Living
a Bhakti Life

YOGA OF DEVOTION

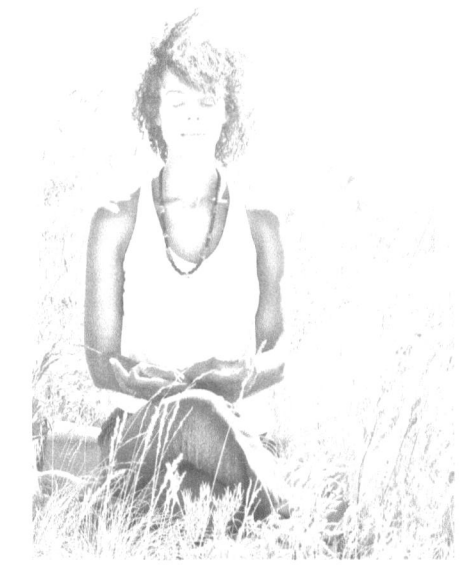

A. R. Pashayan

"People listened because they recognized the words as coming
from somewhere other than the intellectual mind. They seemed
to come from the Source of understanding itself."

Richard Hooper,
The Parallel Sayings - Jesus, Buddha, Krishna, Lao Tzu

iUniverse, Inc.
Bloomington

Living a Bhakti Life
Yoga of Devotion

iUniverse books may be ordered through booksellers or by contacting:

iUniverse
1663 Liberty Drive
Bloomington, IN 47403
www.iuniverse.com
1-800-Authors (1-800-288-4677)

ISBN: 978-1-4759-7033-3 (sc)
ISBN: 978-1-4759-7035-7 (hc)
ISBN: 978-1-4759-7034-0 (e)

Library of Congress Control Number: 2013900219

Printed in the United States of America

iUniverse rev. date: 01/28/2013

Dedication

I dedicate this book to life itself, and the four angels that are constantly teaching me more each day; Donald, Johnathan, Kevin, and Maxwell B.

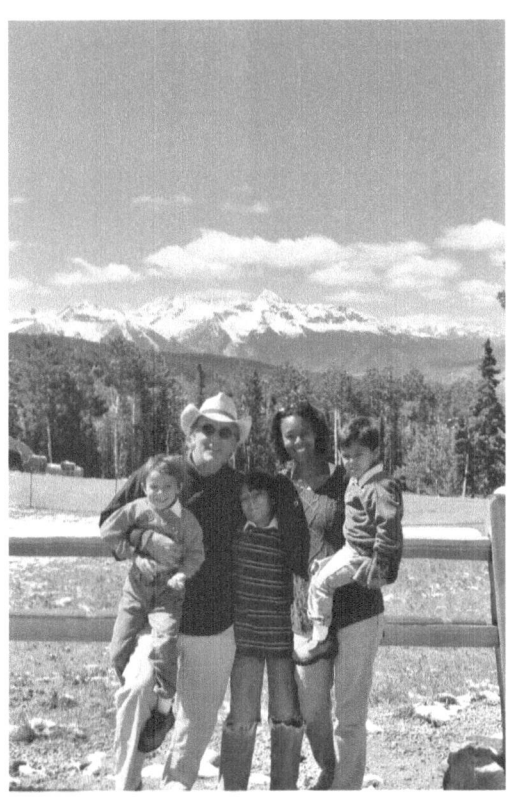

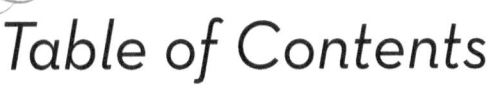

Table of Contents

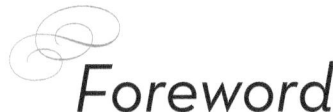

Foreword

Forgive me, I'm a rule-breaker. A foreword is usually written by a peer or professional in the subject matter being written. It is normally someone who knows the author and makes personal statements about how great they are. They tell stories about how funny it was the time they did this or that together, and why the author is such an expert on the topic in the book. My foreword is none of that. Shoot me.

None of us are experts at life. We live it and learn.

My qualifications for writing this book include my daily life growing up in Compton, CA - a poor area with working class people struggling to stay above the poverty level. My days growing up included elementary school where bullets sometimes flew by and gangs were prevalent from 4th grade up. I knew a 6th grader who was head of the Crips....don't know what I'm talking about? Google it. Other parts of my life included runways in Paris and weekends in the Hamptons, go figure? I am an expert at living, and so are you. All of us have a book within, we just don't all have the time or gumption to write it. After living under the roof of a minister/philosopher, I ventured further and broader into spirituality as an adult. I found yoga and began to study various texts on comparative religions. I studied the teachings of Jesus, Buddha, Krishna, and Lao Tzu. I read about dream interpretation and metaphysics. I attended conferences on quantum physics and bought old books by Kurt Vonnegut. I read 'A Course in Miracles' and reviewed the works of spiritual authors old an new. Finally after reading Patanjali's Sutras and the Bhagavad Gita, I realized all the doctrine was the same. The same as what? There is but one Great Spirit and your life flows a lot easier when you learn how to integrate that force into your life. The same as what I learned growing up in Compton.

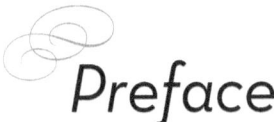
Preface

When you live as I have, you learn to trust in God. There's good, bad, faith, fear and everything in between out there waiting for you to collide with it. There is also peace, love, acceptance, forgiveness and surrender waiting for you as well. My reason for writing the book is to help you find the Great Spirit within and around you, and to help you learn how to navigate life using Bhakti Yoga as a tool.

You are being groomed right now as you read this book. Your interest alone proves that Bhakti living awaits you. But like with childbirth, outside intentions can interfere with the natural path of your spiritual growth. There is no need for wheelchairs to greet the mother in the ER, a laboring woman's legs are not broken. Nor is there need for gowns & masks, the birthing process is natural and requires no special attire. And, decades of scientific evidence have shown that it is far better for women to eat and drink on their own during labor, than to be hydrated intravenously. These outside intentions can disrupt natural birth. Outside intentions can disrupt the natural birth of your spiritual awakening. Instead of wheelchairs and intrusive fetal monitors you experience repetitive behaviors in your relationships or jobs. You experience interference from friends and family, just as a woman in labor experiences nurses that come in frequently and disrupt time for breathing & centering. Bright lights are on and laboring women are not allowed to get up, stand, or move around to find a more comfortable position. You may feel trapped as well in the predicaments of our life.

But then there's oxytocin, known as "the hormone of love" which is at the highest level in a woman's body during and immediately after childbirth. It can swing the birthing experience from pain to euphoria. Oxytocin is like Bhakti, for when you are living a Bhakti Life even painful times (emotional, mental, and physical) are not so bad. Oxytocin has 80 times the analgesic potency of morphine. So does a greater understanding of life. Oxytocin levels for both baby and mother remain high for the first hour after birth... important for falling in love with one another. The euphoric levels of Bhakti also remain high as you continue to practice, making you fall deeper in love with the Divine. Bhakti can be the most spiritual, emotional, physical, and transformative moment of your life.

Your choosing of this book was no accident. For an unknown period of time your spirit has been developing. You have been unconscious of many things that were important to your spiritual growth. Relationships have come and gone making you who you are. And you've always been held in a protective sac, the arms of God-Ishvara-The Divine.

Although it is time for you to be birthed into a deeper level of knowing, the spiritual umbilical cord will never be cut between you and God. Living a Bhakti Life is part of an ongoing, Inter-faith dialog that can birth you into a greater way of being.

May the reading of this book's material give you re-birth of mind and heart so that your spirit is transformed to enjoy the ecstasy of the rest of the days of your life.

Namaste.

Acknowledgments

I acknowledge God, the mother who birthed me, and life itself which continually teaches me through nature and those I am connected with.

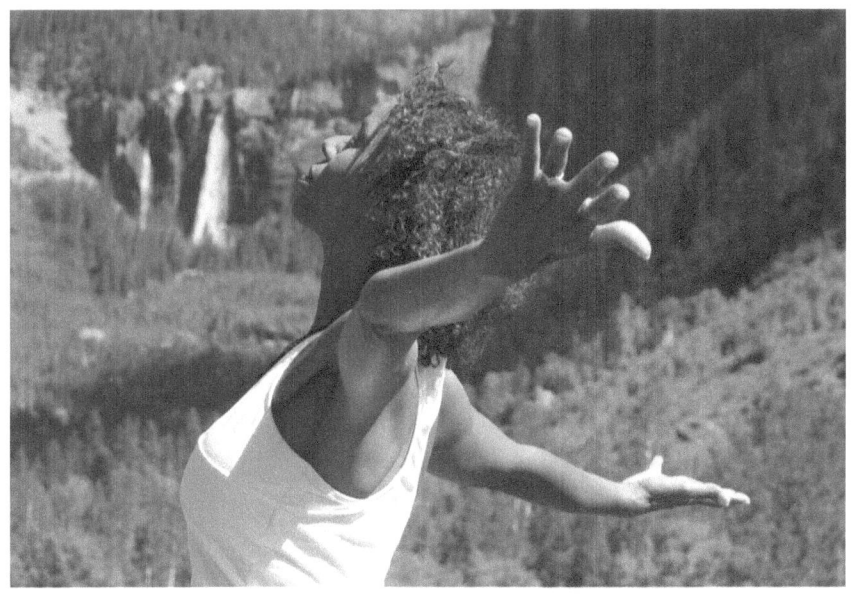

At Bridal Veil Falls, Telluride

Introduction
by Kevin Pashayan - at age 10

Everyone has a special gift, including me. These gifts were give from God for an important reason. My mom has a gift that taught her yoga, love, and peace. My younger brother Max's gift is smartness on things that he's studied and paid attention to such as Pokemon Games. My older brother Johnny's gift has to do with music and Jimmy Hendrix. My dad has the gift of cooking like a chef. My whole family has a gift just like me, but I haven't really found mine yet.

When people have gifts, they have to hold on to it, capture it, and keep it in an imaginary book in their mind. It takes time and patience to grow your gift. You can't fight your gift but you can use it to fight obstacles in your journey. God knows all about your special power and why he gave it to you. You can never hide from God, not even in the depths of the ocean, or in the deepest crevasse. God will always see you.

****

This introduction by my son speaks for itself. It shows that what I instill at home has now made its way to you. This book reflects my desire to inform and encourage you in your yoga practice and spiritual path. This is not only the purpose of the book, but my purpose for being. The significance and impact of learning how to bring Bhakti into your life is crucial to your spiritual growth. In the grand scheme of things, we have not awakened until we learn to incorporate all of life into our practice. The meaning of this body of work is to bring you to live a fuller life with a greater understanding of your journey. The basic premise is learning how to surrender, and how to learn from life all around you. I come from poverty, I am a black woman, my name is Angela, which means *"Messenger from God"*.

Chapter 1
How I Discovered Bhakti

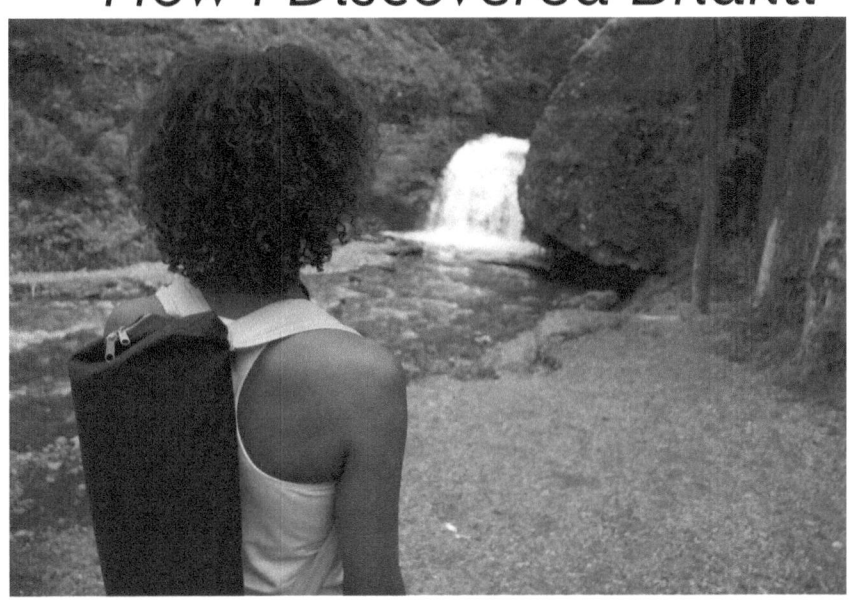

Falls behind Hanley Rink, Telluride

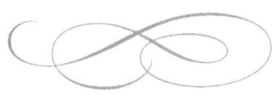

We had been living in Manhattan and the Hamptons when we relocated suddenly to take care of my mother in Compton. It that's not culture shock enough, we had to start all over with our businesses dealing with the left coast....oh sorry, I meant the west coast (smile). With a savings account constantly dwindling, taking care of a toddler and my mother, stress was high even though I was happy to be with Mom. Money use to come easy when I was a Model, working in Europe and New York was a snap and fun at the same time. Now I had to punch into a real bonafide time clock for what seemed like pennies, as I worried about my mom being alone all day. Eventually I was blessed with a great job and my husbands new business took off nicely. However with child number two on the way we were busier than ever. Mom enjoyed the kids, they kept her going. We moved her to Marina Del Rey to enjoy the last years of her life in a different surrounding. She thrived for four years on the love that floated through the house. When child number three was on the way, Mom was on her way out. It seemed like an exchange of life or prana within the family. In August 2003, mourning from the recent death of my mother and celebrating the birth of my third son, my spirit was pinning for space and time to slow down and just 'be'. I knew that something was going to happen soon, either positive or negative. Little did I know, both were occurring simultaneously. Something negative had been happening in my chest, as my heart was pulled in too many directions. I was still grieving the loss of my Mother to whom I was very close, yet my heart was pulled in the complete opposite direction preparing for the beautiful little spirit growing inside of me (my 3rd son). Another emotional tug of war involved my husband, for he needed my time as well as my other two young sons. And don't forget my job......oh and did I forget what we always tend to forget, time for myself. These emotional tugs created a lot of confused energy in my body over my heart, left side = breast cancer.

I moved to Telluride, Colorado on a whim with my husband and three young sons. It was one year nearly to date of my mothers death, and Telluride was intended to be a month long vacation. After 3 days of being there something positive began to take place in my mind and spirit. Protected on three sides by the jagged mountains, I began to feel alive and free from stress and worry. The town, only three blocks long, made life simple. There were limited choices of items to purchase which actually made it easier shopping for everyday items. People were friendly and it was safe there...only one way in and one way out due to the three mountains surrounding the town. A grassy field full of holstein cows (the black and white ones), can be seen at the beginning of town as visitors drive in. Main Street is where it all happens, and no place else. The buildings look like facades from an old western movie. The whole town is preserved by the National Historic Society. Rowdy, one of Americas last real cowboys rides his horse into the Sheridan Bar once a year for a drink. To top it all off, the whole area is surrounded by beautiful nature and perched at 10,000 feet above sea level which makes a blue sky look even bluer if that's possible. I was literally living in the clouds!

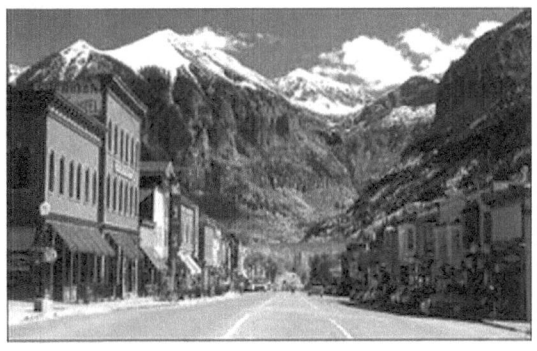

Main St., Telluride

The purity of air and pristine views of the Rockies was like heaven to my spirit, I had found my *"Green Pasture"* from the book of Psalms. God did not have to maketh me lie down, I was ready for it! After 3 days of vacation, my husband and I decided not to return to Los Angeles. I felt a big sense of surrender on that day, that I could leave my ego behind in LA and be content (Santosha) with the simplicity of this town. It was that day I began to learn the Bhakti way. Each day thereafter, another layer of my ego would fall away... and so would my problems. I was on my way to becoming a Bhakti Yogini without even knowing it. I continued to practice yoga and meditation for a year.

Then it happened.

6:30am Telluride, Colorado, 2004

I sat in seated meditation relishing in the bliss of my daily morning ritual. The sweet sound of nothing, strangely audible, filled my soul with a connection to God and to the best within myself. No human presence around me as of yet, all souls in the household still voluntarily unconscious in bed resting in the precious state that is as close to re-birth that is possible. I could feel the presence of the animals in and around my home; the elk and the coyote especially. I filled up spiritually with the mere silence and the most powerful connection I know how to achieve with my creator....as a new method of yoga asana practice arrived in my head. A flood of warmth ran from my Sahasrara Chakra (crown) to my Anahata Chakra (heart). Bhakti chose me.

When it occurred, the experience was likened to those who describe a 'Kundalini Rising' except in reverse. Kundalini Yoga is a style of yoga whereby the ultimate experience includes an electric feeling beginning at the sacrum ending at the crown. The feeing did not occur from the base of my spine to my crown but from a much shorter shorter distance; crown to heart. The intensity of my experience was felt right in the center of my body, physically from the anterior fontanelle (soft spot on crown at birth) through the center of my brain down through my vocal chords and directly into my heart. Unlike Kundalini, I was not altered to a state of non-function but exalted to a state of profound clarity.[1] The skull is made up of 7 bones

---

[1] Medicine Plus www.nlm.nih.gov

that are not joined together firmly at birth. This allows an easier passage through the birth canal. The area where the bones are joined together are called sutures and close naturally over 7 to 19 months after birth. The sutures of the 4 largest bones of the skull create a diamond shape directly above the vocal chords, felt as a 'soft spot' on a newborn. [2]The suture running from temple to temple that connects with the diamond is called the coronal suture. The coronal suture caresses the frontal lobe (the center of thought) and leads to the front of both ears (the center for hearing). The sagittal suture runs from the center of the forehead (Third eye, center for higher purpose) to the top of the Occipital lobe (the center for visual perception). Additionally, the word 'suture' is defined as [3]*the process of joining two surfaces or edges together in a line as if by sewing'*. Complementing this is the sanskrit word *'sutra'*, commonly used in reference to Patanjali's Sutras. The word sutra is defined as [4]*'a thread or line that holds things together'*, metaphorically speaking of the teachings of the sutras. And so we find that the Sutures of our skull at birth have a very coincidental relationship with the power of our thoughts, our programming from God, and the truths of the ancient sutras. All of this to note the importance of the crown of our heads, and to expound that everything regarding our diamond shaped soft spot is absolute perfection from our Creator. Could there be a better way

2 Adam Medical Images www.adameducation.com

3 www.answers.com/topic/suture

4 Sūtra (Sanskrit: सूत्र sūtra, Devanagari: , Pāli: sutta), literally means a thread or line that holds things together, and more metaphorically refers to an aphorism (or line, rule, formula),

to connect with God to receive higher thought, vision, and hearing with the additional purpose of softening our entry into this world? I believe there is no better way, and that the references to the crown chakra in yoga and vedic texts support the crown as our method of connecting to the Divine.

There are yet still other inferences to our point of connection to the Divine being near the crown, think of a '*halo*' as seen on depictions of angels or sentient beings who roam the earth. Even when Bug's Bunny hits his head too hard, the cartoonist illustrates stars or birds flying around his crown perhaps indicating a dis-connect with a sense of wellbeing, or a loss of connection to be well grounded.

The head in relationship to the rest of the body is also thought of as command central. Its the place where all the action occurs to get us moving, thinking, planning, anticipating, reacting, and creating the things we want to do in our lives. It is our '*speak box*' where we can express ourselves verbally to share our truths with one another. It is our vibrational intake center where the highly sensitive eardrum can pick up the vibrations of sounds near and far. It is our olfactory center for smell and taste, which kept us safe from predators and unsafe foods during evolution. And alas our sight, which most often deceives us with illusions that fall prey to our delicate ego. Therefore when this download occurred, something within felt that the crown-throat-chest-heart chakras were the right place for this to happen.

I can best describe the experience as a download of information about yoga postures and their personal meaning, applicable to every practitioner individually. Caps of closure were blown away in regards to the limited manner in which Trikonasana was being taught around the world. Sitting in meditation and basking in an indescribable mental zone, I was keenly aware and astounded at what was being transferred to my mind. I was also afraid, as fear of the unknown surrounded me when I realized that I was not in control. However, my trust in God kept me seated.

Receiving this information felt like a mixture of viewing a high speed movie but with the physical sense of being in the movie. I felt like I was physically in asana practice, while another part of me was the 'watcher' of all that was occurring. My head and chest reverberated with warm ripples of a vibration that was pure as water. These pure vibrations felt like moving energy of light passing through my body in a rhythmic manner, as if the rhythm was communicating something to my cellular structure that cannot be understood in another way. It was as if the vibrations were the message, and sent to a part of me that communicates best through feeling instead of words. A message that speaks the language of sprit.

What accompanied the download immediately afterwards was my own astonishment that I was privy to this information. I thought, "Why was this being imparted to me, a Compton Girl who does yoga at home? Someone *who has not studied under a famous hindu guru, nor ever been to India at that time. Someone who does not wear special head wraps or prayer beads. Someone who does not even practice regularly in a studio. Someone who would be least likely to attract a large audience because famous yogi's are either male or white female."*

There is no black audience in yoga because blacks traditionally think yoga goes against their religion. Since I've never let anything stop me in the past, I let those thoughts go just as quickly as they came to me. I wrote everything down from my mystical experience so that I would not forget the information. I took the rest of the day off to contemplate what had occurred.

That evening during my meditation before bed, the download started up again. I got nervous this time and opened my eyes. I thought, *"Why is this still happening?"*. I began to wonder if something really freaky was going to happen at the end like my head would start spinning around non-stop or something. I went to my husband and explained to him that something strange was occurring during my meditation, and that I wanted him to check in on me often when I started again the next morning. In a totally different mind and place, he agreed *"yea, yea"*.

The next morning I began my meditation again as usual. I normally sit for 60-75 minutes. I heard my husband enter the room to check on me less than five minutes after I began and it comforted me. I quickly found my sweet silence within and the download began to flow once more. It occurred a total of three times over the course of two days, giving me meanings for over 36 postures which I documented at the end of each meditation. With my husband checking in on me, most times I thought I had been meditating my usual hour plus, when actually time had eluded me completely...my husband noting that less than 20 minutes had passed for each of these meditations. *"How could this be?"*, I thought. I felt as if I had been sitting there for hours, allowing this download to take place. It seemed impossible for *less* time to have passed. I knew that the components of experiencing time were different that what most of us believe, and in this case I had actually experienced it.

My spirit was *unified* with the Divine, and I was given information to share with others for healing and liberation of life's illusions that often bring us down. These illusions make us forget who we really are, Children of God, loved and accepted just as we are, and provided for completely. My soul was in a state of surrender; [5]Patanjali's Sutras B.1 V.23 Isvarapranidhanad Va / and B.2 V.45 Samadhi Sidhir Isvarapranidhanat. Both verses mean the same, that a life surrendered to God offering complete service to God's will leads to [6]Samadhi (tranquility of mind). *"Do everything in my Name"* is written in the Bhagavad

---

5 The Yoga Sutras of Patanjali, Translation by Sri Swami Satchidananada 1978
6 The Yoga Sutras of Patanjali, Pg.150 lower 4th paragraph

Gita[7], as are other verses that speak to the nature of Bhakti[8].

During my mystical experience, my sense of time was altered but not my physical being. I felt nothing in my spine or even in my brain for that matter, only as if someone pushed a field of energy through the crown of my head which stopped at my heart and put an internal 'glow' in my chest. I believe Bhakti leaves a permanent mark on the heart of a yogi already inclined for devotion to Ishvara (God). My upbringing and life experiences put me in preparation for this full explosion of surrender.

Many yogi's who yearn for a mystical union with the Divine practice Kundalini, in hopes that they will experience the Kundalini Rising. The actual sensation of my mystical experience differs from Kundalini Rising in an interesting way. Kundalini Rising is of Prakriti (primary matter or the Body). Something physical takes place in the body with Kundalini Rising whereby people have reported intense

---

[7] Bhagavad Gita Chapter 18 By this same love and worship doth he know Me as I am, how high and wonderful, And knowing, straightway enters into Me. And whatsoever deeds he doeth-fixed In Me, as in his refuge - he hath won For ever and for ever by My grace Th' Eternal Rest! So win thou! In thy thoughts Do all thou dost for Me! Renounce for Me! Sacrifice heart and mind and will to Me!

[8] Bhagavad Gita Chapter 11, Shloks (verses) 53-55 after exhibiting His cosmic form, "It is not possible to see me as you have done through the study of the Vedas or by austerities or gifts or by sacrifice; it is only by one-pointed devotion (Bhakti) to me and me alone that you thus see and know me as I am in reality and ultimately reach me. It is he alone who dedicates all his notions and actions to me with a knowledge of my superiority, my devotee with no attachment and who has no enmity to any living being that can reach me". Bhakti therefore, is the only way to the true knowledge of God and the surest way to reach Him. **Bhakti: Unwavering Devotion & Love for God**

electrical impulses moving up and down the spine. People also report being in an altered state afterwards for up to two weeks. My experience was of Perusha (the spirit). Nothing happened to me physically, instead my mind and spirit were vibrating at a fast rate allowing the download to occur. I am taking nothing away from the Kundalini experience, only noting the differences from Bhakti. Bhakti is nearly unexplainable, which is why we have no famous Bhakti Guru's. The closest way to experience it is to understand the practice and practice often. You have to let life teach your heart the rest of the way.

I remained in awe of the experience, then went to share with my husband what occurred. I could not express to him my full excitement. I thought he might get worried and call an exorcist over to check me out. However I did let him know that something unique happened during my meditation, and that I now have a new way of practicing yoga. I left the house after breakfast and went for a long hike to let it all sink in. The hike was good, it gave me time to contemplate the splendor and beauty of this new way to practice. I wondered *"What kind of practice is this? Is there a name that describes it?"*

On hilltop, I looked over my notes written about the postures and began to practice. I cried at the perfection of looking at the past over my left shoulder in a seated twist, and visualizing/creating my future over my right shoulder. Later at home in the full practice, I cried again as I expressed a *'prayer in motion'* through mind, body, and heart in a contemplative way.

My spiritual union with the Divine cranked up my home practice to two hours a day.....not for the sake of vanity but for the sake of working through emotional gunk stuck in my body. It could now be release through this method of asana practice. Through this release came clarity and a commitment to the style of asana I was practicing. My tennis teacher, Sam, noticed the amount of time I was spending on the mat vs on the court and was the first to ask me, "Angela, what style of yoga practice are you doing so much?". I had no definitive answer for him, and his question made me think and led me to research deeper into spiritual texts.

I share these personal details with you in efforts to exemplify that I am a regular human being just like you. I am no more special than you are. What happened to me could happen to anyone. And reading these personal details may jog your memory of times when the Divine may have been trying to communicate with you. Through reading this book, you will be more attuned to subtle nudges from the Divine and find Bhakti within.

I want to share more personal experiences from my upbringing that shed light on the subject matter. Being from the Baptist Church there is a phenomenon that occurs fairly regularly in individuals who have developed a strong personal relationship with God. We call this phenomenon "*Shouting*". It has nothing to do with speaking loudly, rather it is an expression of the body, gyrating and shouting for joy. To viewers at church, Shouting looks like someone has accidentally sat on a sharp tack and discovered their feet are on fire at the same time. I know it sounds comical; however this description can easily be substantiated and seen firsthand by visiting your local Baptist Church, particularly a Black Baptist Church, or searching youtube. When you see someone Shouting, it is initially disturbing. There is physical concern for the wellbeing of the individual who has seemingly been taken over by an unseen spiritual force; their body catapulted out of their seat as if something has suddenly struck their tailbone, proceeded by arching of the back, fast movement of the feet, and vocal shouting. This powerful spiritual force causes one to move throughout the church aisles, running, jumping or walking with uncontrollable body gyrations. Leaders of the church explain this as receiving the *Holy Spirit*. The loving Spirit of God literally visits your physical body, and it is so powerful you've got to get up, move, and shout! The verbalizations range from nonverbal words, to speaking in tongues, to exclamations; *Whew! Oh!* and words of praise like '*Hallelujah, Yes, Praise God, Yes Lord*'. Any blacks reading this will be laughing hysterically right now at the memories of folks shoutin' in church. The physical movements and exclamations are simply a way to release the energy that has come into your body. Shouting usually lasts 1-3 minutes with a cool off period lasting 10-15minutes, as the body returns to its natural state from the experience. Nurses are hired at Black Churches just for this reason. This physical phenomenon calls for medical attention to care for the person's body as it goes into what seems like overload. Nurses of the church are always on hand with fans, water, cool towels and smelling salts, as some bodies get so overloaded with this divine energy they simply faint like a computer shutting down.

I could now definitively answer my tennis teacher's question regarding the style I was vehemently practicing, it was <u>Bhakti Asana, the Yoga of Devotion</u>.

I want to note the impact made upon me from Sri. Swami Satchidananada (deceased in 2002). In his commentary on Patanjalis sutras, he proclaimed publicly to be of no one religion or faith. He was recognized as a Universal Teacher guiding thousands towards Self Realization and serving on Advisory Boards of Peace and Interfaith Organizations Worldwide. He was the Founder of Integral Yoga[9]; integrating body, mind, and spirit in union. While studying the sutras, I found his quote, *"There is another way to find Samahdi, surrender completely to the Divine and do everything in his name"*. Looking further at the sutras, I found references to Ishvara (God) and Bhakti. This is when I discovered the name of the style of yoga I was practicing - Bhakti Asana.

---

[9] http://www.swamisatchidananda.org/docs2/home.htm

May the truth and emotion from the Gayatri Mantra fill your heart with surrender to what you already know is God's love for you.

Om

Bhur Bhuvah Swaha, Tat Savitur Varenyam, Bhargo Devasya Dhimahi, Dhiyo Yo Nah Prachodayat

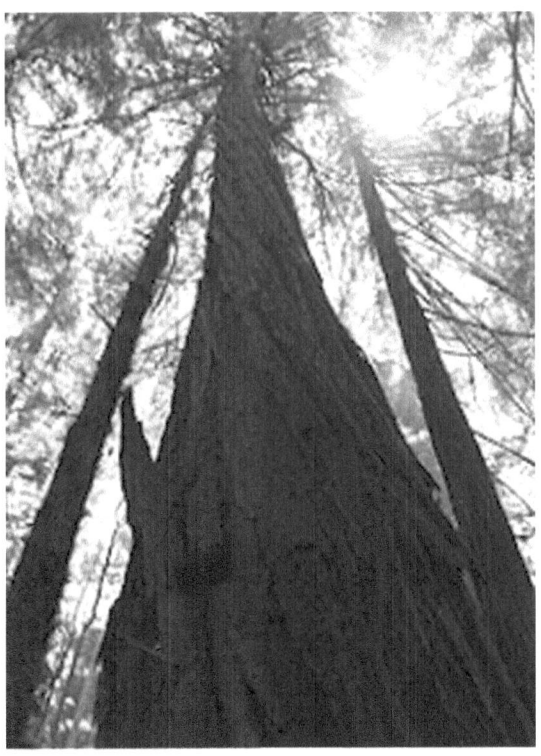

Translation:

[10]May the Almighty God (Om) of the Physical (Bhur),

Mental (Bhuvah) and Spiritual (Swaha).

That one (Tat), the Creator (Savitur) most Adorable (Varenyam),

Gleaming bright (Bhargo) and supreme (Devasya),

We meditate upon (Dhimahi)

That we understand (Dhiyo) your way,

Your light (Yo) (Nah) Enlightens, Guides and Inspires (Prachodayat)

---

10 International Sai Organization www.sathyasai.org

Chapter 2
The Nature of Bhakti

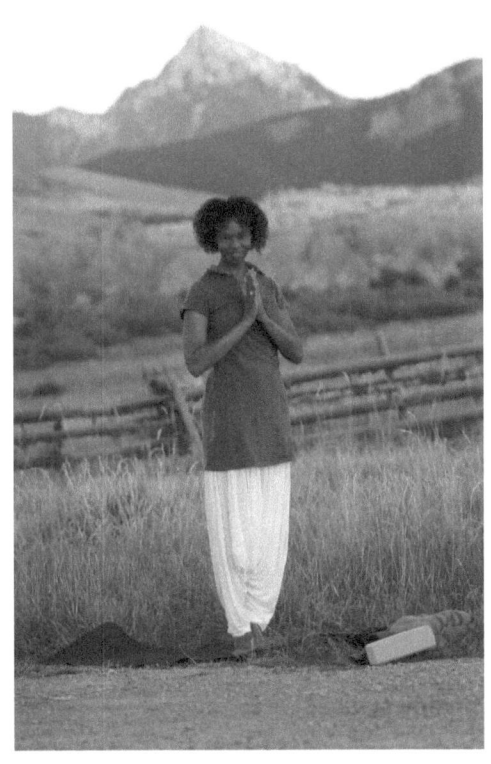

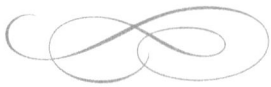

The nature of Bhakti is illusive. It is a way of life that you grow into. I had been emotionally and physically living this life for the two years preceding my union with the Divine. Bhakti is a state of mind that hails from deep within your spirit, and for something that deep to occur there needs to be a protagonist. The protagonist can be a number of experiences but it is important to note that they are always founded in Emotion.

Emotion carries a vibration that leads us back to an unspoken language of the heart, call it *'Emotional Telepathy'*. It's a way of communicating with a higher source, with Ishvara, with God. You always hear people say that 'God is Love', and Bhakti is a way to communicate love to God. Communicating through speaking is wonderful in terms of practicality, however in communicating with the Divine (God) there are numerous ways that express emotional intent far better than the spoken word.

An example of emotional telepathy closest to the spoken word is poetry, like the messages in Psalms from the Bible or a poem by Mary Oliver, Sri Aurobindo, Emily Dickenson, or Rumi. The words of poems are spoken and/ or read with emotion to help you feel the heart of the writer. This method of emotional telepathy uses the left and right brain, satisfying the literal and artistic needs of expression respectively.

Then there is Abstract Art. The emotional content of the artist can be felt in the image itself, the colors chosen, and the intensity of the brush strokes; think of Kandinsky, Miro, Pollock, and Rothko. Somewhere in between poetry and abstract art lies music and dance, both of which engage the body, one vibrationally and the other physically. The pianist expresses tenderness by caressing the keys gently, or power and strength by pressing firmly on the keys. There is even further communication through the facial expressions of the pianist. And of course the combination of notes played as well as the cadence and holding of the notes bear an incredible emotion that is imparted on the listener. Through dance and body expression, emotional telepathy is communicated throughout our whole being. The body expresses the hearts emotion thus increasing the vibrational energy of our intent. Watching the string musicians of an orchestra swaying as they play Brahms Symphony#3, or watching a dynamic Ballet performance can literally make you cry. The tears are birthed not from sadness or happiness, but from an inexplicable emotional place, the place of no words. The beauty of the human form expressing itself in dance becomes a part of the vibration, the vessel of communication. The sound of the symphony without even seeing the orchestra can elicit the same effect by listening with closed eyes. And it is worth nothing that in regards to music, nearly any form of music (rock n roll, R&B, jazz, soul, country, even hip hop) can elicit a strong enough vibrational energy to make you want to jump up and dance; remember, music not only holds the vibration of sound but carries the sentiment of the emotional poetry. Ultimately, the human form surrenders to the power of the unspoken word (the vibe) and becomes one with the message.

This higher form of dialog or emotional communication holds ones feelings and intent as part of the Bhakti union with the Divine. But have you ever felt the intent of a snowflake? An aspen leaf? A river? A mountain? Every natural thing has a vibration and when you are quiet enough you can feel the intent of it all. This unique communication leads to profound gratitude to God, for if the leaves have intent and purpose so must you and every being on the planet. And if the leaves are well taken care of, so are you. And the illusionary death of the leaves when they fall from the trees matches our illusionary human death, as we both simply change forms and continue on to support a new life. I believe that the human spirit finds a new house to live in (a new body) to continue its experiences, and the leaf decomposes on the earth creating essential nutrients for the continued growth of the tree. Feeling the intent of everything around you conjures a deeper understanding of life. The deeper understanding begets clarity, the clarity begets compassion, compassion begets forgiveness, forgiveness begets understanding and unconditional love, which together begets unshakable trust and surrender to the Divine (God) = Bhakti.

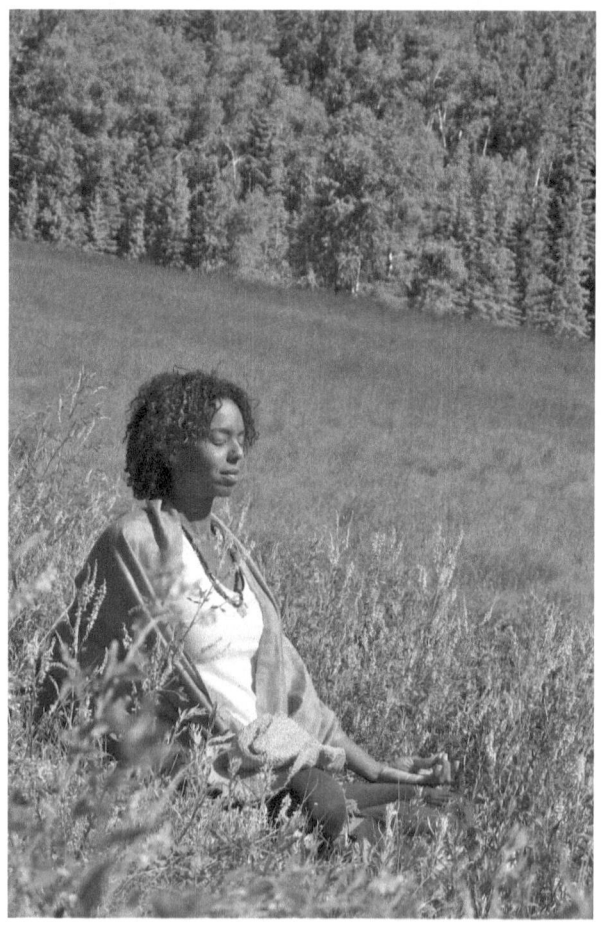

Meditating in nature

Bhakti is multi-layered, it is a way of being gained over time. I found this *'Way'* by walking through the woods of the town where I live, watching the river flow, studying the ease of a red tailed hawks aeronautical glide, and admiring the majesty of a jagged mountain edge. These are all the makings of a Bhakti meditative walk with God. No spoken communication, just the silence of nature and the company of your higher self tapping into the emotional telepathy of everything around you.

Living the Bhakti Way means brining more nature into our lives. How do we integrate this into our busy day? What drives us to even want to pass time in this manner? One way is choice. If you truly want to understand Bhakti, choose to slow down and find the quiet places. Carve out time daily for meditation, or journaling, or taking part in emotional telepathy. The other way to begin understanding Bhakti comes by default; Major illness, loss, or stress. Each carry such a strong emotional vibration, they push us to respond in some emotional way from the heart. However, the response can lead to a higher vibration (going within) or to a lower vibration (acting out), the latter of which pulls you away from Bhakti. Some of us respond with a quiet contemplation of Life & God; going within. Others respond by yelling and screaming at everyone around; acting out.

Nature itself is not the single answer to finding Bhakti, it is simply a doorway to show you the profound perfection of God. Illness is another doorway. Both can leave you wondering what this whole thing is about, or you can be transformed toward seeing the profound perfection of it all. Out in nature one realizes there is nothing to do, no place to be,no church pew needed, no reason to worry, no need for fear, no place for grudges. One realizes that anger, resentment, and stubbornness are so incredibly ignorant it is embarrassing. The leaf is never pissed off at the branch, nor are the roots mad because they are hidden underground. The birds don't hold a grudge against the fish, neither do they worry all day about their next meal. And the snowflake is never disappointed that its unique, one of a kind shape not only goes unrecognized, but even gets pressed out of shape and stepped upon. Talk about true liberation....it seems that a sparrow is more of a Jivamukti (liberated one) than anyone else! In the hospital bed, patients begin self pity with "Why me?" and then begin to contemplate their predicament. Having a broken leg typically won't lead to deep contemplation, the injury has to be something that might lead to death. The human spirit quietly goes through a conscious life review trying to figure out what went wrong causing the illness. What usually comes up are memories of emotional pain or anger. Experiences and memories of harsh criticism can curl fingers and the spine leading to arthritis. The body takes the criticism as a personal attack and curls downward searching for a new way to become grounded. Back to the hospital bed, the correlation becomes clear in the patients mind, although not shared with the doctors or anyone else. A patient with eye problems may realize that they've seen enough of life and need a break. Someone with stomach issues may not be digesting life very well. Overall, the intent of your body and the path of the illness can speak loud and clear when illness is serious.

The nature of Bhakti is using emotional telepathy to hear, see, and learn whats going on within you. And whatever that might be, it's not worth getting sick over. Let it go and find freedom in surrender. Surrender what? Surrender your life, your journey, your worry, your fear, your ego – and let life carry you instead of struggling against it. Allow experience to guide you, trusting that whatever occurs – life is meant to make you a better person. Surrender your need for control, your effort to be perfect, your idea to have it all, your perception of 'Why me'. Let go of your resentments and judgements of others, no longer caring that your brother ruins every Christmas. He too is in your life to help you grow. Drop the fear of what may happen tomorrow...it's not even here! Surrender your ego and the obsession to loose the extra two inches on your waistline. Shed your likes, dislikes, and accept who you are and where you are in life. Surrender your heart to God, that you may be an instrument of peace and love among mankind in whatever type of work you do. Surrender to the truth that you are a Child of this Universe[11] with an omnipotent parent who has already taken care of your every need. God is the ultimate expert at emotional telepathy; you think it, he gets it!

You can call God whatever you want; Allah, Kali Durga, Krishna, Jesus, Buddha, Mohammed, Krishna, Atman, Brahman, or Ishvara as noted in the sutras. He is but one great spirit no matter the name. I can call you Tom, Fred,

---

11   Faith Rivera – "Child of this Universe" Lil' Girl Productions / Spiritual Songstress & Writer

Lisa, or Susan and you would still be 'you' right? We are all looking for a personal relationship with the ultimate higher source. It is our culture that applies the name to that source, and it is our ignorance that alludes us to believe there can be no other name for this higher source. Some find Jesus in church, others find Brahman surfing waves, still others find Atman through their paintbrushes, Buddha on a mountaintop, Krishna at Kirtan, Mohammed at a special meal. And I find God through my Bhakti practice.

If we were all meant to find or Creator through one method, why are there so many flavors of the same message of love, peace, compassion, and understanding? A powerful creator could surely make it so that every nation and every culture uses the same spiritual name to call him. But this great spirit gave us free will to create, express articulate in our own way. This freedom has caused some of the greatest wars.......and some of the greatest works of art. It's a matter of spiritual maturity to accept that God is God everywhere. Our variety of practices and/or worship may be different, but God remains the same. The parallel sayings of Christianity, Buddhism, The Upanishads, and the Tao are collected nicely in a published manuscript[12] by Richard Hooper. The jest of all four texts is: <u>Be nice, be content, trust in God, and check-in with God</u>. Checking-in takes us back to emotional telepathy or Dhyana (from the 8 limbs of Ashtanga Yoga), using feelings of the heart to communicate with God whether in prayer, meditation,

---

[12] Richard Hooper, 2007 – The Teachings of Four Mystical Traditions; Jesus, Buddha, Krishna, & Lao Tzu / Sanctuary Publications

taking a walk, cleaning the house, making dinner, in church, or on a prayer rug. Being 'nice' includes Ahimsa (non-harming) to other living things around you, and this is a big discussion for another book. Being 'content' (Santosha in Patanjali's Sutras) is rooted in the finding happiness in the way things are. Cicero says, *"If you have a garden and a library, you have everything you need"*. Lastly, "trust in God" is what leads to Samadhi (union with the Divine or Bhakti). It requires full surrender of your ego, of thinking that you know better than God how to guide your spirit through life. However, it does not mean acting irresponsibly for your welfare, waiting for a magic chariot to sweep you out of trouble. It means surrendering the old way of thinking, being, acting, living, reacting, and loving. It means using emotional telepathy, it means Bhakti.

Chapter 3
Ishvarapranidhana:
My life in Telluride

"And when it flows, it is coming from a place of Surrender"

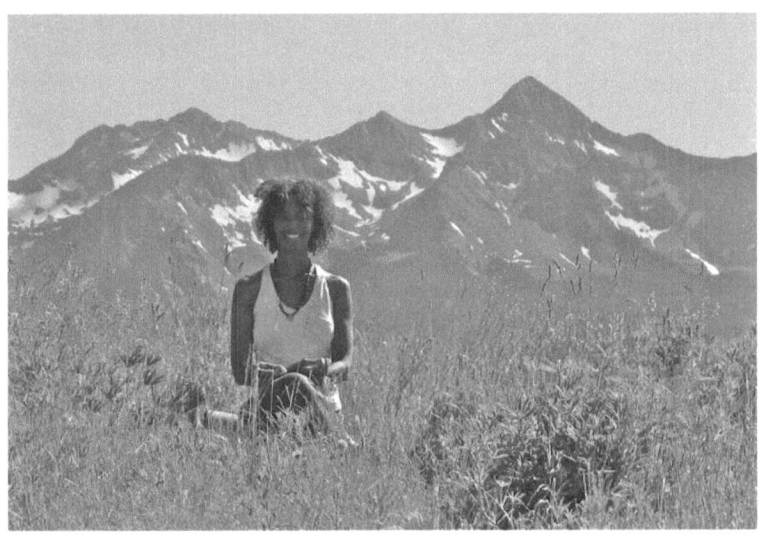

Meditating near Wilson Peak

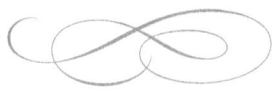

I did absolutely nothing in Telluride. Burnt out from the city, it was my time to heal. My husband understood. Though I did nothing, something 'did' me and it was Bhakti. Each day I rose and watched the most incredible sunrise over Bridal Veil Falls. The mountain peaks in Telluride are very jagged, unlike other mountain resorts. It was these jagged formations that lead my eyes to gaze more intently. The sharpness drags you in to look deeply for more of nature's treasures until you begin to see crevices, shaded areas, and snow in hidden pockets. You begin to see life around the jagged edges and know that they are home to animals, plants, snowflakes, wind, and rain. You begin to see the majesty of the Mountain; its strength and power although it simply sits stationery. You know that some of the sharpest edges have offered the gentlest shelter to some living thing. And you begin to contemplate God's perfection in the balance of power and grace. And this is only sunrise.

The remains of the morning for me would include Meditation, Yoga, and then breakfast. The Meditation began around 8am lasting only five minutes the first time. I worked my way up to eight minutes and finally ten whole minutes! I felt this was a huge accomplishment and it took two straight weeks to get to this point. Each morning I sat and thought about no-thing. Many times I was interrupted by my grocery list, household chore musts, current news images still floating in my head, not to mention the loss of sensation in my knees and feet from sitting. All of that was all right, as I held no judgment and just kept at it every day. By the third week I was up to 15 minutes and within two months I was up to 40 minutes. What does this feel like? It feels like heaven in that all things of any matter go away and you are left with a deep sense of silence. In this silence you find the essence of you, your spirit with its highest vibrations hovering at your heart. You cannot find it with your eyes open, and it takes a while to reach it even with your eyes closed. But when you do, the bliss of loosing the Prakriti (physical self) for those next few moments makes you not want to return to the world of matter. You feel so free and at ease that nothing else matters – No Thing Matters. I can stay in this place easily for an hour, and it was in this place or in this state that I began to find myself merging with God. I could sit with God, ask questions, acknowledge God's miracles in nature, share the beauty of the mountain through images stored in my mind, and speak of God's grace without using man-made words. I used my heart. Bhakti was developing.

After my morning meditation I would take breakfast, usually in silence. Each step of preparing the meal was a visceral treat. My eyes enjoyed the shades of brown within the flakes of oatmeal, the sound of the milk pouring onto the dry cereal, the bowl; a vessel that holds it all together and neither asks or receives the merit it deserves. The perfect round shape of the orange and the citrus scent from the rind. It seemed I was continually learning about God's perfection as I cut the orange in half and saw the most beautiful and bright orange color gazing up at me inviting me to partake of its nourishment. The steam from the coffee pot pierced through the air almost in a bewitching way, the aroma a treat for the sense of smell. And finally the treat for the palette, each bite of breakfast tasting incredibly delicious.

My day after breakfast was more of a mix of experiences flowing between duties of daily life and rendezvousing with God. There was computer time to check e-mails, reply to mail, pay bills, clean the house, and all the usual stuff that we all do. However, there was a break for me around 1pm after lunch. This was me & God's time again, and it in-

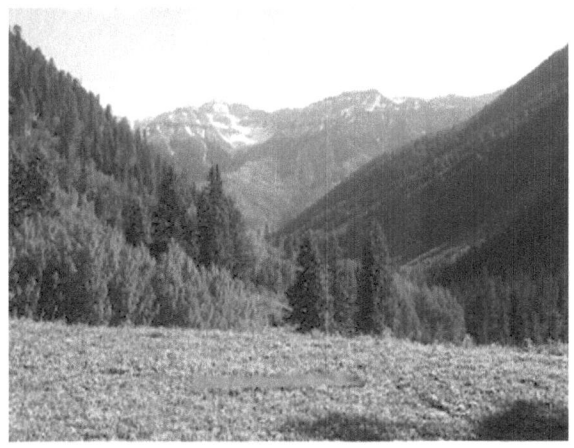

My mat, my spot – Bear Creek Plateau

cluded a hike through the woods. My favorite place to hike was and still is Bear Creek Canyon in Telluride. My afternoon time with God was equally as powerful as my morning meditation. I would stop early on and admire the aspen's creating a winding path up the mountain, the sun shining down on parts of the path reminded me of the bright times in my own personal path. There are locations all along Bear Creek to veer off and sit along the creek which is more like a river. Snow from the top of the mountain feeds into the creek creating a bustling flow over rocks and fallen branches from an elevation of just under 10,000 feet. The trail is four miles total with an elevation climb of 1040 feet from bottom to top and there are beaver dams and wildflowers all along the path. I would always find a place to sit along the river for a short

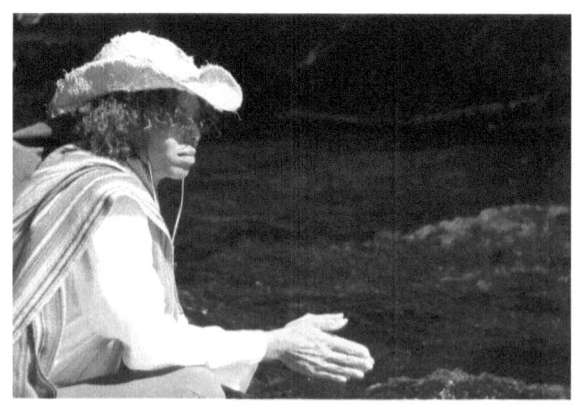

On the River Trail

meditation, then continue up to the flat plateau for a few more yoga stretches, finishing my hike at the top where the waterfall would pound five feet to my right and down the mountain into the creek. Hiking a trail like this becomes a walking meditation. Seeing the power of nature surrendering onto itself becomes an acronym to mankind's potential relationship with God. Bhakti was developing further within me.

My evenings consisted of family time, sometimes joyful and sometimes tedious; dinner, homework and bath-time for my boys, bedtime stories, and finally my "rendezvous with God" to seal in the day. This evening meditation was again up to 40 minutes and consisted of a mental review of the day and gratitude for all it brought. I acknowledged the souls connected to me and my journey, grateful for my friends and foes. I dwelled in the seat of forgiveness for taking so long to see God's beauty in literally everything. I stood before God in line for service. Bhakti was upon my spirit.

April is mud season in Telluride, and I remember being on vacation with my family; a week in Cancun, Mexico and another week in the small town of Tulum. I continued my yoga practice and meditation daily, switching out walks up the mountain for swimming and kayaking in the ocean. We stayed at the Westin and were given a gift from the hotel for our stay; certificates for food, spa, or tour. While my family enjoyed food by the pool, I enjoyed a Spa Treatment. The treatment I choose was an ancient Mayan Purification Ritual which included a body scrub with healing plants, therapeutic incense, special sage brushing to purify the spirit and massage. It was during the massage that I went into meditation and noticed for the first time a round, purple, moving abstract image on the inside of my forehead between my brows (my third eye). This image is difficult to explain, though I will do my best to describe it; it begins as a round purple circle and then begins to morph into unusual shapes, bending around the edges to the point of collapsing into what looks like a black hole. Somehow the black hole seems to regenerate the energy of the purple circle and the circle reappears from its crunched in shape again. I watched the shape intently, trying to understand its form and collapse. I've tried to extrapolate if there were letters or words being formed, but there is nothing more than the expansion and contraction of the circle, kind of like the arbitrary formations of clouds drifting in the sky. Once it gets going, I cannot tell at which point it is contracting or expanding, it all seems like one. I knew that this was some kind of Bhakti gift, another way to connect with the Divine. But I did not know how to use this gift.

Point here is that the lifestyle in Telluride, Colorado provided the foundation for me to receive Bhakti. The simplicity and time afforded me to slow down and listen to life. Many of you reading right now, long to slow down. Some of you have found your balance yet still crave more down time. I'm here to tell you there is no way to find this peaceful lifestyle if you don't make it happen yourself. No one is going to provide it for you. No one. Its up to you. Retreats are a way to let go for a week or two, and I suggest planning them twice a year as well as maintaining a meditation practice at home. It's the best way towards living a Bhakti Life.

Chapter 4
Virabhadrasana III:
Share your Gifts

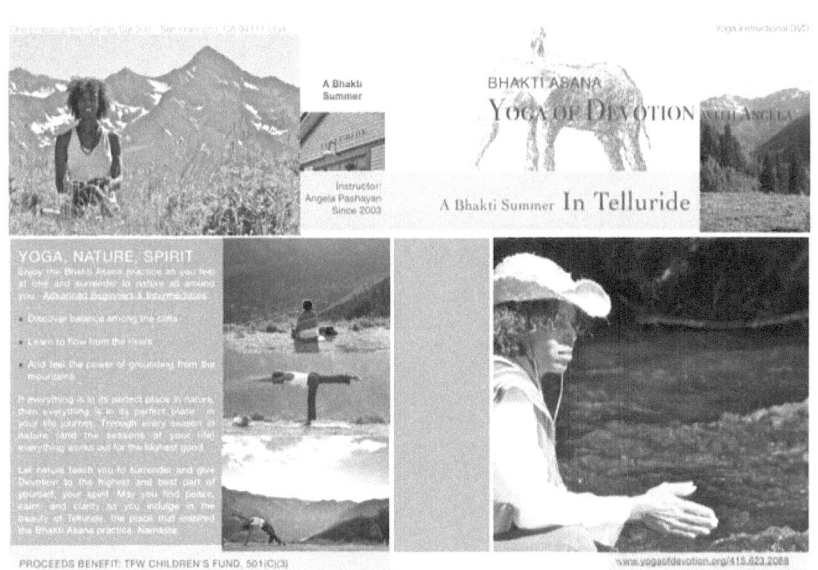

DVD cover

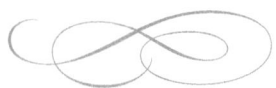

After practicing Bhakti Asana for nearly two years and burning away the old residue of life's experiences, Warrior three was one posture that I realized I had no spiritual meaning for. I practiced Warrior three daily, and I just thought perhaps there were some postures that did not have deeper meaning. I received meanings for the basic postures and I could build from there. Then one morning from Warrior One pose, I arched my back letting my arms fly open to the sides. My chest and heart were completely open towards heaven, and I felt a deep sense of letting go while being open and vulnerable to whatever was to come my way. I brought my hands back to prayer at the heart (Anjali Mudra) and moved into Warrior Three....... at which time I got another download:

"Together we are Spiritual Warriors. Take all the gifts I have given you, move forward and share those gifts with the world."

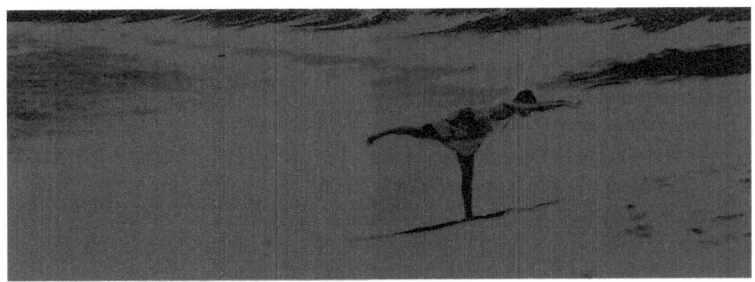

Vira III/Warrior 3 in Kauai

This was the last download and it occurred *not* in seated meditation. I was moving through time in a physical way and at a level of consciousness that was deeply meditative. My whole Bhakti Asana practice was in essence, a meditation. It was a *Moving Meditation*, a physical surrender and body prayer. My level of consciousness may not have been as deep as in seated meditation, but the elements of focus and heartfelt intention to let go were present. In my asana practice, I released my mind and ego regarding getting the pose. Instead I aligned the downloaded affirmations with my body's physical capabilities in each posture.

And so, I had received my final Bhakti affirmation, a gift with a double meaning; the sentiment of the posture, and instructions for me to get out and TEACH this Bhakti Asana yoga practice to the world. Ironically it was not what I had in mind for my future.

If you know history well, you will recall that nearly every enlightened soul struggled with their destiny. In other words, no one wants to do their job. It's actually quite interesting how we would rather take a simple menial job, than do something spiritual that requires our vulnerability and potential failure to be appreciated. If we are delivering mail, we will be understood and appreciated. If we are filing papers or preparing reports we will also be valued. But if we are delivering a spiritual message.....there's no guarantee people will even hear you out. Do you think Moses really wanted to climb Mt. Sinai, a dry and jagged rocky mountain that was smoking at the top? He even convinced his pal Aaron to climb with him for a while so as not to go it alone. And what was Moses going up there for anyway? In a meditative state he was told to climb the mountain to receive the commandments of God to share with the world. Don't believe in God? It's ok, there's plenty other examples like Dear Prince Siddhartha who was raised in complete luxury whose only choice to find bliss was to renunciate of all his wealth and ultimately become the Buddha 'awakened one'. Do you think that preachers really want to commit every week of their lives to preaching, meetings, bible study, etc? Do you think that authors like Louise Hay and Wayne Dyer raised their hands as kids affirming to take the adult job of modern day Prophets? Try Gandhi.....oh yes, he really enjoys starving – NOT! Martin Luther King, Jr., anxious to speak against racism during a time when blacks had fewer rights than dogs. And there's me, a black woman from Compton spreading the word about Bhakti before it was mentioned by any famous guru or western yoga philosophers.

If you look deeper into history, you will find that not only were the chosen ones unaware of their higher purpose, but seemingly misguided as their life circumstances took them through an Instant karma cycle as they were being groomed for their jobs:

- Moses, alive only because he was put in a basket on a river, and raised in royalty when he was a jew (the despised culture of slaves)

- Dr. King, why could he not have been born White and speak about the injustice of racism?
- Louise Hay, sexual abuse, broken home, illness
- Wane Dyer, orphan, alcoholic
- Prince Siddhartha, rich and meant to be a Mighty Ruler to live in luxury
- Gandhi, a privileged Indian sent to school in London to be an attorney yet escaped to a life of poverty

Jesus was the only one completely aware of his higher purpose, yet his life seemed to encompass every setback under the sun; illegitimate conception, stressful prenatal life, born in a dirty barn, poor family, as an adult his work was hard labor (carpenter), and he befriended whores and lepers as a spiritual man. Kurt Vonnegut even goes on to say, [13]"If Jesus were alive today we would kill him for the same reason he was killed the first time, his ideas are just too liberal".

I fall under the category of those like Robin Hood, common but noble. However, I am not in the global spotlight nor am I a household name. I'm just a young black girl from Compton with a message, preferably delivered on the yoga mat. How quirky of a choice for God to chose me to deliver a message to a predominantly all white audience of yogi's. If I were at least a Female Caucasian I might stand to get a little more attention in the yoga community. If you only knew how many times I reached out to others for help with no response (including Gaiam and Russell

---

[13] Pg. 22, Armageddon in Retrospect, Kurt Vonnegut 2008

Simmons). No harm felt, if Jesus can take being hung on the cross I can certainly take being shunned by big whigs. I am honored to be the *pioneer* that I am as a female and a part of the Afro-American Community.

Contrary to the illusionary quirkiness of God choosing me, my life has prepared me with "instant karma" for my spiritual job as it did life for the aforementioned spiritual leaders. Did you know that Moses' name literally means "drawn out of water"? Wayne Dyer can speak compellingly about the Way (The Tao) only because he has experienced 'loosing' the way. Buddha taught renunciation of riches with the understanding of how difficult it is to turn away from wealth. And in fact, he ended his teachings with this quote, [14] "There have been many Buddha's before me and there will be many in the future – All living beings have the Buddha nature and can become Buddha's".

And so my life preparation and karma includes being born nine years after my brother and two sisters. This means developing maturity early on. This also develops independence and the ability to be alone with ease. The near ten year gap caused me to see things differently than my siblings, not to mention my parents were very different people by the time I was born. My name is Angel..a which is defined as; A female Angel and messenger for God. My father is a preacher, philosopher, and community leader with excellent speaking presence. My late mother was the star of any show, beaming love and a gorgeous

---

14 http://online.sfsu.edu/~rone/Buddhism/footsteps.htm

smile to everyone she met be they homeless or the Mayor of the city. She was and school teacher and owned her own day care center named Children's University. My birthplace is Compton, California. My upbringing included the philosophy that I could do anything in life; just think it, act as if, and know it's on the way. My teachers were divorced parents, older siblings mistakes, church hypocrites, infidelity, the Crips and the Piru's. Then there were lessons in foreign travel, the jet set life, vanity of fashion, marriage, entrepreneurship, motherhood, heart failure & compassion, breast cancer, yoga, nature, and San Francisco's diversity. All of these life experiences I take into my heart moving from Warrior One to Warrior Three, committing to share my gifts with the world and lead others to understand the message of Bhakti.

Chapter 5
The Garland of Life, or the Noose of the Journey?

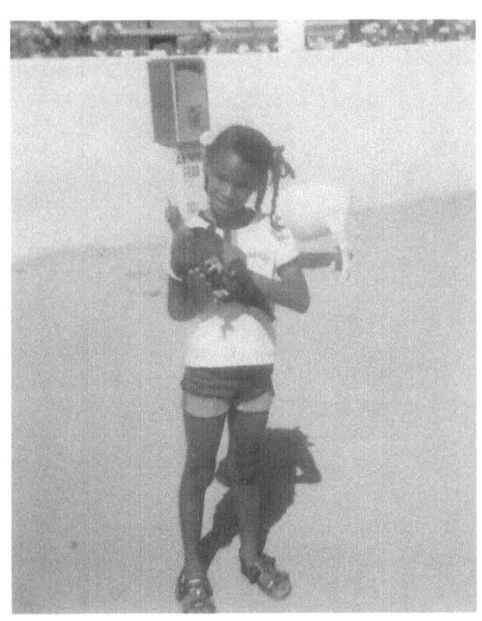

A. R. Pashayan as a girl

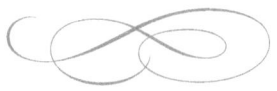

After the Warrior Three experience it became clear that I was to teach. Promptly dropping this notion from thoughts, it picked itself up from wherever I dropped it and found its way back into my head every time I took to the mat which was twice a day - "*You need to teach, why aren't you teaching, hey ever thought of teaching, you mean you are not going to share this asana method, others will benefit from your teachings, cant you see you have been given this method for a reason?*". Talk about monkey mind! When I received the download I felt like I received the Garland of Life in all of its splendor. However, I was now beginning to feel the noose of the journey :(

I finally gave in, but with lots of back talk to the Divine; "*How will I do teacher training with three children at home? Where is the money coming from for this training? How will I find the right teacher? How will I find students who want to learn this strange new method after being licensed? What is the name of this method? What will my husband think? Will yoga students study with a black chick? Where is this all taking me personally?*"

I was honored to have received the method (The Garland), but reluctant to begin the journey of sharing it (The Noose). Have you ever put on a certain color, or got a new haircut, or wore your clothing differently and felt awkward? This was me in my skin every day. How in the heaven was I supposed to pull this off in a yoga community that focuses more on alignment of the body than of the soul? A community that cares more about loosing inches than loosing spokes in the wheel of Samsara's?

My download of Bhakti Asana postures came to me through my heartfelt Surrender to the Divine, a surrender to let the universe/God use me as needed for the Highest Good. I thought the highest good would involve my family, my neighbors, a stranger or a child in need...but I was not counting on serving a larger audience like The World. God thinks big and I thought I did too until faced with the worldwide job of sharing this message. I surrendered in my practice, and now I was following through to carry out the job that was given to me. In the book, The Mind of Jesus, there is a quote that captures what I felt the Divine was communicating to me:

[15]"And God was saying; *The priests have lost me, the wise men have lost me, the people seek me and cannot find me. It is our task to tell men of me and bring them to my love.*"

---

[15] The Mind of Jesus, pg.7, William Barclay, Harper & Row Publishers, New York 1961

As fearful as this was to accept, It became easier to walk my journey after being blessed with a beautiful dream. The dream took me back to my childhood, about age five, sitting in the front row of my father's church watching my mother lead a song with the choir. The dream was actually a real memory of mine. I felt comfortable and it felt good to see my mom singing deeply from her heart, a song that us church folk knew so well. She wore blue and had her choir robe open in the front. She stood on the red carpeted platform, not far from where the assistant preachers and my father sat. It was always hot in church so there was light perspiration on her face. The church parishioners stirred when she approached the microphone and the introductory notes of the song were played on piano by my Aunt Bobbie. They stirred again with anticipatory joy of the feeling they know their souls would feel hearing my Mom Billie sing *"Nothing Can Turn Me Around"*.

At five years old, I knew this song well from hearing it during rehearsals and from Billie practicing at home. I sat alone on that front pew, older siblings somewhere else in the church. I watched her intently as she began singing:

"Nothing can turn me around,
I've started for Heaven and I cant turn around.......
I want to hear, him say, when he comes, on that day,
Servant Well Done!
And that is why, I know, that
Nothing,
Can turn, me around"

This dream closed after the song ended. When I woke and recalled the dream, I knew from that moment onwards that I would wear the garland of life and fulfill God's work throughout my life journey, never to turn back.

First step was finding a yoga school to become teacher certified. I knew I'd find no school of Bhakti, so I just looked for a school that appealed to me. After searching the internet I learned that 200hrs of training was required which came to a solid month of instruction time unless I split the training up into individual weeks. I also learned that the cost of training ranged from $3000 to $6000 depending on the quality and variety of instruction. I had an old periodical (Elephant Magazine), in which there was an article on an Iyengar yoga teacher named Tias Little. The periodical was over three years old but I kept it because I was moved by that particular article. I looked at the article again and noticed that Tias had a yoga school in Santa Fe, New Mexico. Not only was Santa Fe one of my favorite places to visit, it was only a five hour drive from Telluride! I meditated on this as a possibility for my training, then searched the web for the school. I found a 30 day training beginning May 15th and I could live at the training facility which was an incredible Buddhist Center in the foothills of Santa Fe along a river.

Speaking to my husband about all of this was next. As I began the subject matter, he was not surprised at all that I would want to become a yoga teacher. We discussed that he alone would have to care for our three sons during two of the four weeks, then drive to a vacation rental in Santa Fe where I would join them for the last two weeks of my training.

Lastly was the issue of the money, training was nearly $5500. I needed a job. Over the next few days here's what happened: In meditation I asked for a job, I looked in the classifieds of the Telluride Watch Newspaper, I made a call, and I got a job. It was that easy. I was hired to work for the Zoline Family at the Telluride Institute as a part-time Marketing/PR Specialist. It was temporary work and it ended after three months as I earned just enough for the training. The training itself was fulfilling, as Tias is one of the more philosophic teachers which made me feel at home because my father is very philosophic. The teachings included studies in anatomy, physiology, poetry, sanskrit, meditation, chanting, nutrition, ayurveda, asana, vedic history and ethics. The setting was ancient pueblo style housing with multiple building and meeting spaces separated by gardens and walking paths. A central kitchen was where we not only took our meals in the Buddhist tradition of silence, but a place of seva where we all volunteered to cook, clean and prepare the dining hall. The whole experience was meant to be.

While there, some of my favorite times were in the stillness of meditation with our teacher Elisa. She was graceful and oh so peaceful. We were with her every morning at 6:30am for an hour, sitting. Often we would begin with no words at all, just sitting in the quiet. Then Elisa would begin speaking quietly to teach us the days lesson on meditation. I'm taking this time now to emphasize the power of quiet, the power of stillness. And I must note that everything about Elisa is peaceful. I have never met anyone who exudes such a peace naturally.

She taught us one chant in a call and response fashion that will never leave my heart and mind, Kayena Vaca. I cried when I learned it, as it's meaning went straight to the heart of Bhakti. Written in sanskrit below, it's meaning dedicates everything, every cell, every thought, every act, every breath, every part of oneself to The Divine Consciousness. In hindu tradition, Lord Narayana is lord of the waters. Water is a symbol of consciousness which flows everywhere, including both the high and the low places on earth. Water flows with ease, no struggle, purifying whatever is in its path. Water heals and cleanses, washing away what was and starting anew. Water caresses and neutralizes, creating comfort and pleasure. And with our bodies being made of nearly 70% water, we are a part of that great consciousness. We are a part of God. May Kayena Vaca touch your heart as it continually does mine.

Kayena Vaca

Kay/ena Va/ca , Manasen/driy/airva

Buddhy/atmana/ va, Prak/rteh Sva/bha/vat

Karomi Yad/yat, Sakalam Paras/mai

Nara/yana/yeti, Samar/payami

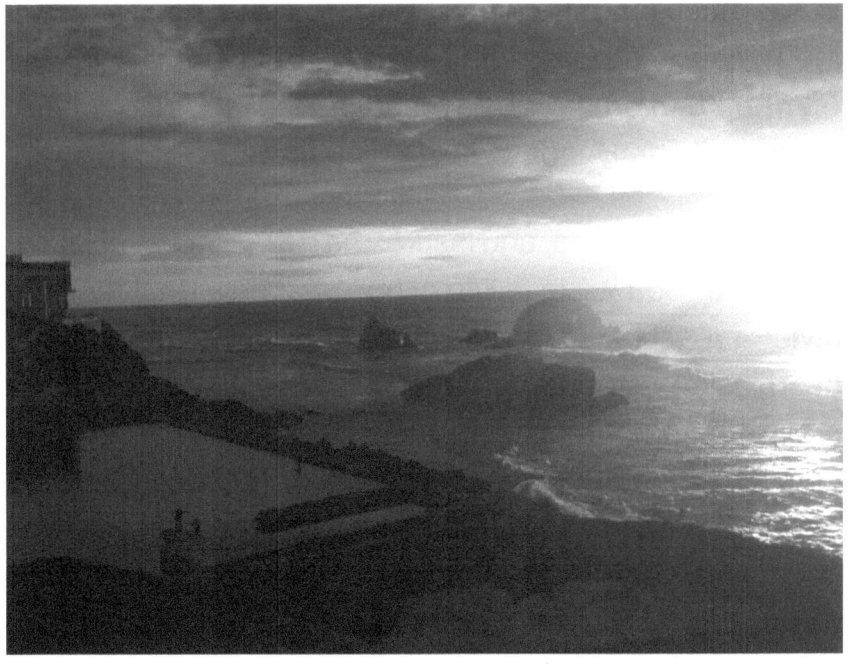

San Franscisco Sunset

Whatever I do with my body, speech, mind or senses;
intellect, self, or natural disposition/constitution – all
of these I offer completely to the Supreme Being of
Consciousness (The Divine).

After my training in Santa Fe, I returned to Telluride and formed a non-profit organization for my work. I decided to give back with every asana to the God that revealed such a beautiful practice to me. Everything fell into place with training, teachers, family, and finances. The Garland of Life felt good!

Now for the Noose....

It was after the bliss of the training that I began to feel the noose.[16] "*Nature puts to work the acting frame, but Spirit doth inform it, and so causes feelings of pain and pleasure*", The Bhagavad Gita, Chapter 13.

Registered, certified, and insured as a teacher I sent letters out to the yoga world telling of my great new Bhakti Asana style of teaching. Whoever read these letters was either dead inside, too busy to care, or fearful of supporting the odd messenger (me). I received no responses or negative responses. I started a weekly class in Telluride that went nowhere. I had a 3:30pm time slot and those of you who teach know what a lousy time slot that is. I gained some private clients, but I thought, "*I should be teaching to the world – not three persons in the world*". I reached out to the spiritual community at Hay House and Mishka who run large conferences. I asked to teach and speak ...... for

---

16 The Bhagavad Gita, Translated by Sir Edwin Arnold, Ch.13 pg.139, Watkins Publishing, London 2006

free! No takers. In meditation I began to ask *"What was the purpose of giving me something I cannot share?"*

A short time later I felt the urge to go to India, the place where many of the texts I learned about were written. I booked a trip and thanks to some strings pulled by my Jr. High School buddy Lateef, I flew business class! In India I experienced the colors and sounds of life itself. I was in the south of India, in Kerala. I saw poverty yet felt the bliss of living at the same time. I practiced yoga and had extensive ayurvedic treatments daily organized by a doctor who could read my whole life through my pulse. Not once did I choose the treatment I wanted, he decided what I needed.

During the day I went to local places and watched humanity; how they lived, worked, communicated. I looked at faces, smiles, taxi drivers, animals. I watched children and their mothers. I was feeling he pulse of India. I became friends with a local and visited his family. They offered me the best chair in the house, then just sat before me staring with smiles on their faces. The house was two to three rooms total (not bedrooms, just rooms), and there were eight people sitting before me. None of this was that strange for me, remember I'm from 'the hood', and if the Blacks haven't done it already the Mexicans surely have. I come from a place of understanding, not from a place of judgement. A roof is a roof, and family is family. My friends home was not be big, but there was love present there. I was falling in love with India, and it was good for me to be there to help me find clarity in my purpose of receiving the Bhakti Asana Practice.

I asked my friend if he could arrange for me to ride an elephant and that same day I was atop of one, riding through the streets of Kerala. What a strange sensation being on an elephant with cars and trucks whizzing by right next to you. Even more strange experiencing the trucks at eye level! I thought, *"What's a Compton Girl doing on an elephant in the middle of the street?"*

My time on the elephant was short, maybe one hour. I asked if I could take another day with the elephant in a quiet location. I wanted to *'be'* with the elephant, not ride it or work it. It was arranged and set up for two days later at 6am. That morning was mystical, as the sun rose heating up the village roads I watched the mist rise into the day.

At our location deep into the jungle foliage of a nearby village, I wandered around to survey the area and be at one with the nature around me. It was 6:30am and the villagers were now coming out towards the grassy central area of the village. The elephant arrived, not the same one as before. I walked to meet it. I spent time quietly getting to know it, intuiting its feelings and sharing emotional telepathy. I made my intentions clear, that I just wanted to be with it exchanging a non-verbal dialog of oneness. As time progressed, I climbed upon the elephant and made my way into a few yoga postures feeling the support and strength of the animal beneath me. It was an amazing feeling, the tenderness of the morning and the gentleness of the elephant carrying my intention.

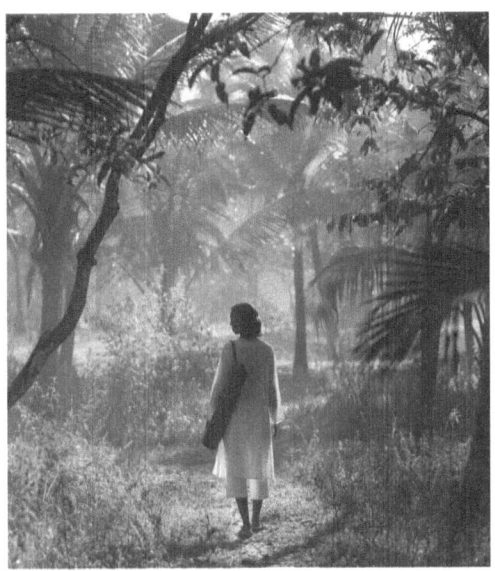

Dawn in Kerala, India

At this time, I did not know the hindu meaning of the elephant Ganesha....that Ganesha removes all obstacles in its path with nothing stopping it. God has a way of communicating with us, and if we don't pay attention we miss his divine directions. For it was shortly after the trip, I believe that the elephant experience was telling me that nothing could stop me from sharing my gift with the world. That if I just continued to move slowly and gracefully, I could remove all obstacles in my path. I could raise vantage point of life, looking out from a higher perspective. And I could take my time with all of this, as I've never seen an elephant in a rush. My foundations are solid, grounded, and my power comes from within - just like an elephant.

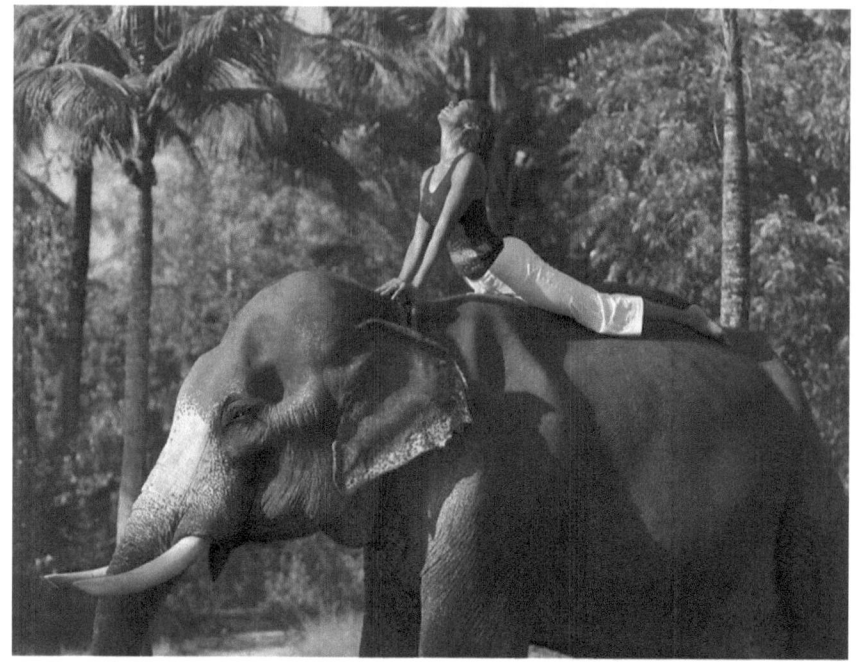

Updog – Kerala, India

A few months later, something began to stir. It was my sense of grounding, literally. For some reason our landlord was suddenly in a rush to sell the home we had been renting for three years, and he wanted us out quick! It was November, the worse time to find housing in Telluride due to the ski season. It was also 2007, and in hindsight our landlord got wind of a coming recession and was told to sell now!

We found a temporary rental by the grace of Steve Cieciu, a dear friend realtor. Rentals were getting so difficult to find in general so we talked about making a move out of Telluride. We also wanted our kids to get a broader perspective on life. We decided to move either to Santa Fe, back to East Hampton, or to San Francisco. After checking out schools and overall lifestyles in all three locations, San Francisco was our choice. And for my work in yoga & spirituality, San Francisco was a great location!

With the Noose lifted, we moved and I ventured into the yoga community. I began teaching at two studios, subbing at others, and trying to connect with the people at Yoga Journal Magazine. I opened a business office downtown, a physical yoga studio in the Mission District, and beefed up my website. I volunteered for various organizations. I networked at events. Everyone I taught or met was deeply moved by my explanation of the Bhakti practice, yet my yoga classes were still small and not financially fruitful. I was struggling to stay open and soon I was struggling to meet my own personal needs. The effects of the recession were hitting as early as mid 2008. I had decided that funds for classes would be used to help children in need, taking a salary only when there were sufficient funds. My husbands' business was declining also. The Garland once again began to feel like a Noose.

By 2009, the burden of the journey was becoming too great. The recession was in full rage and dragging me and my family through the mud. I had to let go of my pride and find humility in resources like the food bank, Medicare, and low income bus passes, and food stamps. I distinctively

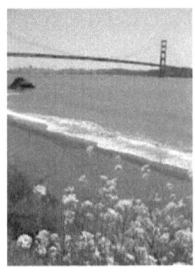

Golden Gate from Kirby Cove

remember a period of six months where we went without coffee, a period of nine months without foil or lunch bags for my children. I remember the same ransit looking sponge we had to use for the kitchen dishes, which also had to be used to wipe the floor because the mop died. I budgeted carefully the use of toilet paper, *borrowing* any extra rolls I could find in public restrooms. I used dishwashing liquid in the washing machine to clean our clothes for nearly eight months. My kids shared one cut apple between the three of them for for lunch with peanut butter sandwiches (no jelly, it was not in the budget). And there came a time when I had to give up teaching a yoga class at Glide Memorial because I could not afford the $3.00 to get there and back. We soon discovered other resources like Free Hot Lunch for children in school and the Dollar Store for household cleaning items. These are all things you don't know when you have never been financially unstable.

I realize now that the noose of the journey and the garland of life are one in the same.

They should not be thought of as different things. There is no need in trying to separate the two, for they are one. If you take nothing more from this book, take this; Bhakti means Surrender and whatever is hanging around your neck, whether it is a garland or a noose, you must surrender to the burden or integrity that comes with it in order to fulfill your karma.

I kept going through life on a day by day basis. I gave up trying to *"make"* something happen. I found the simplicity of existing good enough for the day. I became deeply grateful for what I had and appreciative for what I lost. I let go of worry and released all doubt about my wellbeing because each day I was poorer than the day before, and yet the needs of myself and my family were met. My cup may not have been running over with abundance of the tangible, yet there was no end to the overflow of spiritual growth and love in my heart for life as it taught my family humility, gratitude, and understanding. This is not a tribute to me, I'm writing this for you to see how life becomes your teacher.

"The teachings are more important than the teacher."
Richard Hooper

Chapter 6
4 Steps to Bhakti:

1.) Personal relationship with God
2.) Yoga: the Inter-faith Dialog
3.) Meditation & Music: The Climate for Spirituality
4.) Nature & Compassion

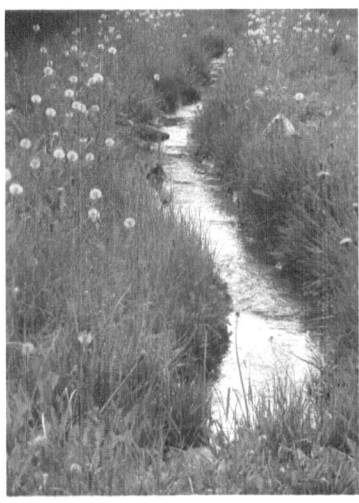

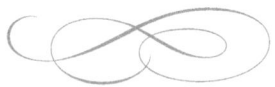

1.) Personal Relationship with God

If Bhakti means surrender and devotion to the Divine (God), then you must have a personal relationship with the Divine that cultivates a level of trust. Why would you surrender to someone you do not trust? How is this level of trust gained?

When a mother gives birth, the first hour afterwards she has the highest level of Oxytocin (the love hormone) she will ever have in her body. The same is true for the newborn baby. As the mother is holding the baby in her arms after childbirth, the Oxytocin is at work bonding the two eternally. But there is another bond that goes unseen, the bond that began at inception between God and the embryo which goes even farther back to the bond of God and the mother at the time she was an embryo. God is our creator, the ultimate mom.

The main evidence of this bond usually shows itself when we need the help of God, like in childbirth. We cry out "Oh God, help me get through this". Further evidence of this bond is seen during tragedies when we cry out "God, help us". Something within us knows when to call upon God. It's as if we automatically know when a job is meant for God and no one else. This bond is eternal, as is a mother's love for her child. It does not matter what the child does wrong, the mother still loves her own. There is also a bond between father and child, but without the Oxytocin.

When someone loves you no matter what you do, who you are, what you accomplish and what you don't.....that's unconditional love. When you are loved unconditionally, you trust that person with your life. You have no problem going to that person and saying "Guide me please, I leave it up to you because I trust you". Often, that person knows what's best for you and can direct you back on your path. As a child we surrender daily to our parents, but particularly our mother; flopping in her arms and crying for her to make it all better. When we burn our hand after having been repeatedly told not to play with matches, we realize that mom knew best. When we date the wrong person or choose the wrong car, mom just waits on standby to help us when everything falls apart. She's always there for us. *So is God.*

If we can trust mom with our lives, we can learn to trust God.

Begin by looking deeper into your life at the times when mom was not there to help. Look at the times that you narrowly escaped a car accident, or made it to a meeting just in time. Think of the occasions where you could have lost your lease, or could have fallen from bad footing. Who was there helping you? Was it blind luck.....all those times? There are so many other occasions that you are not even aware of; You were stopped by slow granny crossing the street to be averted from a speeding car two blocks ahead. You didn't get into Columbia University because you would not have met your spouse at UCLA. You didn't get that great job because you would not have learned to be grateful. Take a moment and journal the times in your life that were pivotal. Note the good, the bad, and the ugly. Dissect those times and find the lesson. Dissect those times and find God.

When you begin to see God working in your life, you realize that good or bad, God know's what is best....just like mamma. Mamma's got eyes behind her head, so does God. God will sometimes let you learn the hard way, just like mamma. And even if you call mamma a bad name, she will forgive you just like God. As you journal those intense times in your life, take some time and talk to God-Ishvara giving thanks for the hard knocks and the gentle nudges to keep you on track. Begin to talk to Ishvara every day asking for guidance to see clearly what is needed to bring you closer to the alignment of peace and love. Ask for signs and then really take the day to look for them. Sit in meditation and talk to Ishvara using emotional telepathy, or just listen. I often ask questions and wait for the answer.

As you get to know God, you will begin to enjoy the relationship with this all knowing divine entity. You may not always get the answers you want, and sometimes you will but not on your time. For Ishvara is connecting the dots to many lives at once, so your getting a new home is intertwined with the personal growth of the seller, the broker, and perhaps the neighbors. It's not all about you, but at the same time, it is. It's not always the beginning of something, sometimes its the end. And if you have a family it gets even more complex because the life experiences can be for the spiritual growth of your spouse or your child.

It all comes down to trust. Do you trust God? Or do you think the moon and the stars are held in place by Donald Trump? Yes there's science to help us figure out lots of the mysteries of our existence - but in the end science still cannot explain *why* an atom reacts the way it does, only how an atom will react....and even that is not 100% predictable! There is a higher intelligence that is our source: Hindus call it Ishvara, Muslims call it Mohammed, Christians call it God, Atheists call it Fate, Poets call it Love, Scientists call it Intelligence. If you trust that gravity will hold you in place this very minute, then you already trust in a higher power on some level.

When you have a personal relationship with God, you can let go of fear, hatred, jealousy and worry. You know that everything is in order for your growth towards unconditional love. Whether you practice yoga, or meditation does not matter with Bhakti. It's about trusting that God is with you, like a teammate. It's about seeing the face of God in each face you meet. It's about serving others when you can in simple or extravagant ways because that's what God does for you every day. When I had cancer, I trusted God and was OK with dying or living. I did get the lesson of my cancer, which I will share with you in another book.

We as yogi's talk about re-incarnation openly, yet still struggle with day to day life trusting our journey. We are not running out of time, and the object of life is not to get it all done. When you are dead there will still be something in your in-box. Bhakti allows you to relax and live, trusting that all is well.

Build your relationship with the Divine and begin the Bhakti Life.

2.) Yoga: the Inter-Faith Dialog

In all of your life experiences, do you think your body has been a bystander? Do you believe that your body has not been affected at all? Your body is more involved than you realize. What you experienced is a part of your mind, body and spirit. It makes you who you are. For example, if you experience something unpleasant it gets stored. The question is, where? It obviously gets filed in your memory (the mind), but what you don't realize is that it also gets stored in your body. Emotional experiences like to get stored in large areas of the body, like hips and the back. These areas are huge compared to our limbs. They offer strength and plenty of area to lodge in. Experiences also get stored in your Spirit, causing you to have hypersensitivity to certain situations.

The body, mind, and spirit are storehouses for all our experiences. This is how we learn. Some experiences get embedded and decrease our flexibility, not just in the body but in the mind and spirit as well. We become stubborn, a form of mental inflexibility. We become afraid, a form of Spiritual inflexibility. We become stiff, a form of physical inflexibility. All of this is meant to protect us from harm. Becoming rigid is the same as becoming compact and strong. Becoming flexible is the same as becoming loose and potentially vulnerable. A body builder's form is tight with muscles and posture inward spiraling, while a yogi is just the opposite - loose and ever expanding outward.

Look at your own posture - stand in front of a mirror sideways. Notice if your natural position is slightly rounded forward and inward. This is the most common stance of most who live in modern civilization. We are tired, run down by the systems we have created, and slightly guarded for good reasons. We don't live up to the sexy standards we see in magazines or films, we don't have stock in Apple, and we can't even afford a decent two week vacation.

On the contrary, those who live naturally are off the grid. They have no electric bill to pay, rising with the light of day and sleeping when the sun goes down. Living off the land with organic farms as their back yard they wear no makeup or fancy clothes, and feel no pressure from films and magazines. They work the land and get grounded from their hands in the earth. They observe nature in the production of the harvest. They have plenty of downtime, with no need for a vacation in Hawaii. They have meditative time during cooking, planting, walking, bathing.....it's all built into their daily life. And....their posture is broad and open, not rounded.

It is not a bad choice to live in modern society, but it is not a good choice to allow life to bear heavily on the body, mind, and spirit. The combination of exercising all three is crucial to maintaining overall health and wellbeing. No matter your religion or culture, Yoga is the inter-faith dialog that can free your being from embedded experiences. Bhakti Asana (Yoga of Devotion) is a tool for transcendence. Freely choose from the "menu" of postures following your urges. Your spirit choreographs its own sequence, tuning into your inner needs. Yoga of Devotion is meditation or prayer in motion.

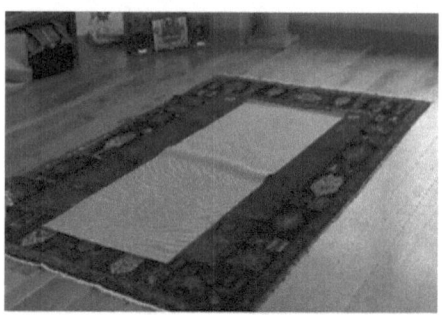

Home practice

To live the Bhakti life, find your own flow and follow your urges to create your own yoga sequence. Respect and trust your body's needs. It know's what needs to be stretched. You can start by lying flat on the mat, knees into the chest and twisting them to the right as you look towards the left. With arms spread wide, let the pose testify to the different directions we are pulled every day in our lives. Lye there, don't rush to switch sides. Use your mind to release the twists and turns of life, let it go through the twisting of your spine. Breath and imagine the twists and turns of life leaving your body, mind, and spirit. No need to figure out those twists and turns, surrender the reason for them and trust that Ishvara-God-Life has your personal growth in mind through every turn. Now switch sides and rest there a while. Coming out completely to continue your practice, or stop there and enjoy savasana. Remember that savasana is not for snoring, its for contemplation of the posture itself (Corpse Pose). From a Bhakti perspective this means letting every muscle go, including those in the face, mouth, tongue, and jaw. Take savasana as a time to feel the freedom of doing nothing, just like a corpse. Bhakti living encourages you to explore savasana, allowing the surrender of all your self judgements to sink into the earth and be recycled into something new. Know that your divine source is with you: God, Ishvara, Mohammed, Allah, Brahman, Jesus, Buddha. Let it go, clean your slate, and roll over to your side coming up and awakening to a new birth, a fresh you.

The inter-faith dialog with God continues throughout each posture, until you can practice without a tear and with the fierceness of knowing that there is a tender and perfect Divine Presence within you guiding your life. Yoga of Devotion (Bhakti Asana) takes the symbolism of yoga postures as concrete representations of inner spiritual disposition. Savasana (Corpse Pose) in itself is highly significant, opening the body and being vulnerable in a position of trust with open palms as a gesture of readiness to receive. Carolyn Cronk and Rev. Nancy Roth teach Yoga for Christians in a similar way in their book, A New Christian Yoga. It can be difficult getting through just three postures, so take it easy and don't force anything. This is Asana for self cleansing, a purification process. When I began practicing this way, getting through a full Surya Namaskar (Sun Salutation) was all I could bear: Taking in all of my life experiences (good and bad), swan diving into the day, then dropping for Chaturanga to lower my expectations of others, pushing through and looking up to the Divine for my power, finally to restore myself back into the balance of life. The list of Bhakti Asana Postures and their meaning is printed in the back of the book. The postures that are not listed are for you to build your own meaning into, using the root meanings that are listed.

3.) Meditation & Music: The Climate for Spirituality

By becoming more balanced in the body, mind, and spirit one becomes more receptive to God. Meditation is a way to quiet the mind and become centered. When in that state of focus, you will find yourself more in contact with your spiritual nature. Here, you can collect yourself and create an atmosphere of inner peace, a deep calm and harmony within the soul. Here, you are preparing yourself for an experience with the Divine.

In Meditation, the breath is essential - for this is the very source of energy that animates your spirit. Long, deep, slow, full breaths is the key. Find that rhythm on you own. Each body and ability is different. Each person's lung capacity will vary, as some of you will breath fully but at a faster pace than others. No worries, please don't try to be the ancient yogi who can control their breath better than a blue whale. Be you. Your breathing will elongate becoming longer and smoother as your mind settles and as you practice more. Your heart rate will lower, your brain waves will drop, your nervous system will be calmed and your brain will develop a heightened awareness creating the climate for spirituality. The union of a still mind, body, and spirit jump-starts the process of a deeper union with ourselves, others and all of creation. A physiological high is often what is felt when in deep meditation and afterwards.

Certain things can enhance your practice, including;

time, space, comfort, and attitude.

a.) Time:

Find a regular time to meditate. One of the purest times is early morning before the world awakens. Wake up ten minutes earlier than usual and meditate in bed initially, using a pillow under the back of your buttocks for support. The bed is not the best place to meditate because it is often soft and not good for seated postures, however its a realistic way to begin. Keep a robe or blanket nearby to keep you warm. You will eventually move your practice to another spot. The Bhakti Life is about devotion, and a second meditation time in the evening is necessary. Again, ten minutes as soon as you finish working is a sound beginning. Drop everything at the door and sit, releasing the days events through your meditation. I promise you will feel better for the rest of your evening.

b.) Space:

Find a space and claim it for those minutes in meditation. It does not have to be the same space, although there is nothing wrong with creating a space with an alter, etc. The Bhakti Life is liberated, and no space if off limits.

You can come home in the evening and meditate at the kitchen table. If you do not live alone, people will buzz around you looking for snacks, getting water, etc. Just let them. They will soon realize that you will not break until you are ready, and leave you alone. You may choose to meditate outdoors in the mornings during the warmer months. Stake your claim no matter the ant or dragonfly that wiz by you. Finally, you may prefer to meditate indoors in front of an alter. Create *YOUR* alter. Whether it holds a statue of Buddha, Shiva, Jesus, or a single stalk Daisy it's your choice.

c.) Comfort Clothing:

This one is real simple....no tight clothes. Meditation is tough enough to do without your clothing pulling at your body to distract you.

d.) Attitude:

If your mind gets distracted, or shall I say *when* your mind get distracted, just keep at it. We live busy lives and it takes a while for our minds to settle. The ten minutes of meditation are just enough to get you in the habit, but not long enough to get you to that deep wonderful state which is your goal. Don't be dismayed, let your disappointment go and just do the work. Soon you will feel the urge to meditate longer; you'll find that fifteen minutes feels better, then twenty, and sixty for some. Remember, we are all different.

Music helps create the climate for spirituality as well. It's all about the vibrations that move through the body. We are water, 60% as adults and 85% as infants. Water moves with the slightest touch. We are moved with the slightest touch. Our water make-up is two-thirds Intracellular fluid (25 liters) and 1/3 (15 liters) Extracellular. Transcellular fluids are not even counted, they are 'third space' fluids contained in organs: cerebrospinal, gastrointestinal, and ocular. The brain is 70% water and our lungs are 90% water. The lungs have the highest percentage of water compared to any organ in the body. I believe there's a reason for this. The lungs are the intake for prana (life force) and the lungs surround the heart. The vibrations of music move us to sing along, clap, and dance. Coupled with the right lyrics or arrangement, the vibrations of music will touch the hear in a profound way.

If you cannot meditate in seated silence, let your meditation be the attentiveness to spiritual music. Find music that uplifts you or fills you with emotion. It can be chanting or instrumental. It can be Asian, Hindi, Middle Eastern, or from the West. As long as it truly moves you is what counts. No faking is allowed; don't play the Gayatri Mantra if it does not touch your heart and likewise, just because James Brown moves you doesn't mean your are to play it twice a day. Search iTunes or visit a music store and create *YOUR* mix. Listen to your mix in the morning while you dress or eat. Listen to your mix in the evening. Ten minutes is fine, you don't need to listen to the whole CD.

The Bhakti Life needs to be fed with meditation and/or music. It creates a climate for spirituality within the cellular structure of your body, brain and heart. Body counting for 65% water, Brain 70%, and Heart 90%. A study done in 2009 by Dr. Andrew Newberg, Radiology Department at the Hospital of the University of Pennsylvania [17] showed brainwave activity of those spiritually moved during the deepest moments of faith. Those moments were precluded by inspirational messages or prayer. The frontal lobe of the brain was less active or *"not in charge"*, God was. There was a surrender or letting go and letting God. The study showed a higher response in the frontal lobe when the cameraman was not present in the room with the participants, and the highest response when Spiritual Music was played. The responses were higher than those of monks and nuns recorded during meditation.

Find your mix, find your heart and find your Spirituality.

4.) Nature & Compassion

There is something within my past lives that still drives me today. My love of travel, horses, and being a protector of those in need have been with me all of my life. I sat one morning reading a book I purchased after visiting the Himalayan Mountains near Nepal. The book references the Grand Trunk Road in Pakistan; 27 miles through the

---

[17] http://www.pbs.org/wnet/religionandethics/episodes/july-17-2009/faith-and-the-brain/3597/ - Dr. Andrew Newberg - University of Pennsylvania Brain Study

rocky foothills between Peshawar and the Afghan border, also known as the Khyber Pass. The writer speaks about the Kachi Gahi refugee camp of over 1.5million Afghans displaced after the Soviet Invasion. He asks a local Pakistani how he feels about the costs of taking care of the refugees and the answer was beautiful, *"We're all the same people"*.

compassion prevails. The statement of this local Pakistani is true, *we really are all the same people.* The sooner we realize this, the sooner compassion will grow all around the word, and from within. For every molecule of air that gets pushed in one direction, there is a reaction that occurs in the environment. For every human being that helps another human being, there is an emotion that is released. What is released (due to air or human emotion) is real, and continues to affect the environment of plant life or human life. Its a ripple effect.

The Bhakti spirit has compassion for every living thing. To live a Bhakti Life means to acknowledge that everything on earth is here to support something else. Everything is interconnected. The exchange of carbon dioxide from trees and carbon monoxide from Humans is a prime example. And how ironic is it that cow dung is what helps produce the best produce! Then there's this incredible world of teamwork interconnectedness of ants, bee's, and other small animals who work together for a greater good. Everything works together for a greater good......except us humans. We try, but ego usually gets in the way with things like greed, selfishness, jealousy, pride and fear. To live a Bhakti life, one must cultivate enough compassion within that there is an urge to help another being - not and urge from intellect but from the heart. A Bhakti Yogi knows that the emotion released from an act of compassion is absorbed into the collective conscience of the world, and spread to others who have that Bhakti spark within them.

The Bhakti Life also includes precious time with nature. Nature is where its at, it's where to go for answers. It's often the choice place for meditation or yoga. A simple

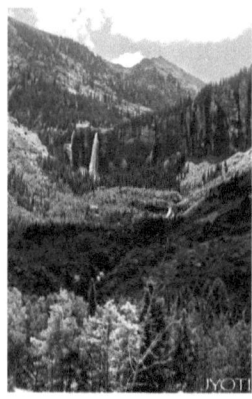

Falls at Idorado, Telluride

nature walk provides the time to go inward and notice your planet teammates; leaves, trees, birds, dead tree trunks, streams, rocks, ants, flowers. Once out in nature, you can stop and meditate in an open field and feel the vastness of space around you - or sit by a stream and see how the water continues to flow whether it has to curve around a rock or drop over a waterfall. You see the rocks on your path and realize that with each step you are receiving a massage on the sole of your feet. And if the ants or the rocks or the stream were not there, something would be affected.

Go deeper into the Bhakti Life and take the same amount of time contemplating the larger partners of life; the mountains, the blue sky, the sun, the valleys. What are they saying to you? What do they teach? The blue sky can teach us a variety of things; the vastness of our world, the limitation of range of colors we can perceive, or the incredible protection our ozone layer provides. The sun speaks to the skin on our faces encouraging the pores to open and let in vitamin D and K. The mountains and the valleys provide perspective for us to climb and view, or take refuge in their protection. To live a Bhakti Life, get out into nature alone. As you become friends with nature, you learn compassion. You begin to see the interconnectedness of all.

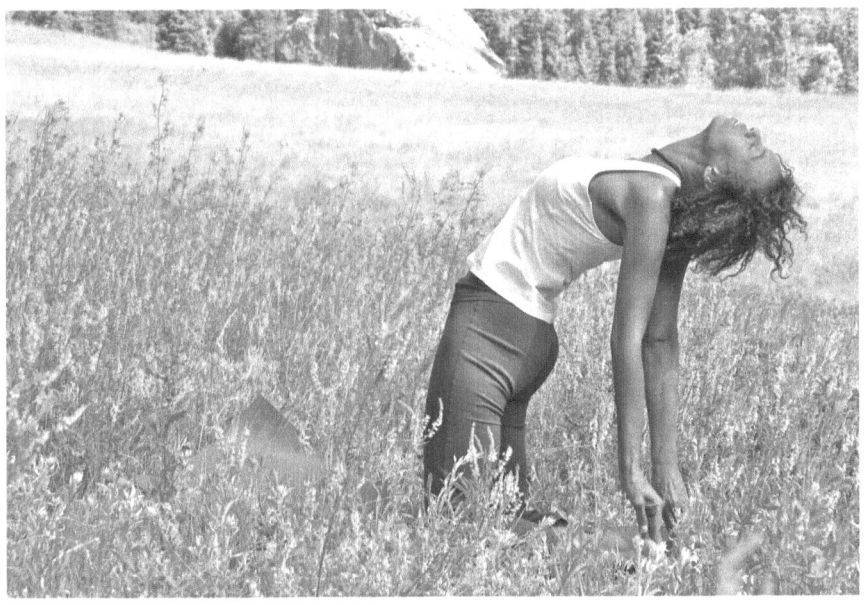

Backbend in nature, Idorado – Telluride

Chapter 7
One Nation, With Liberty and Yoga for All

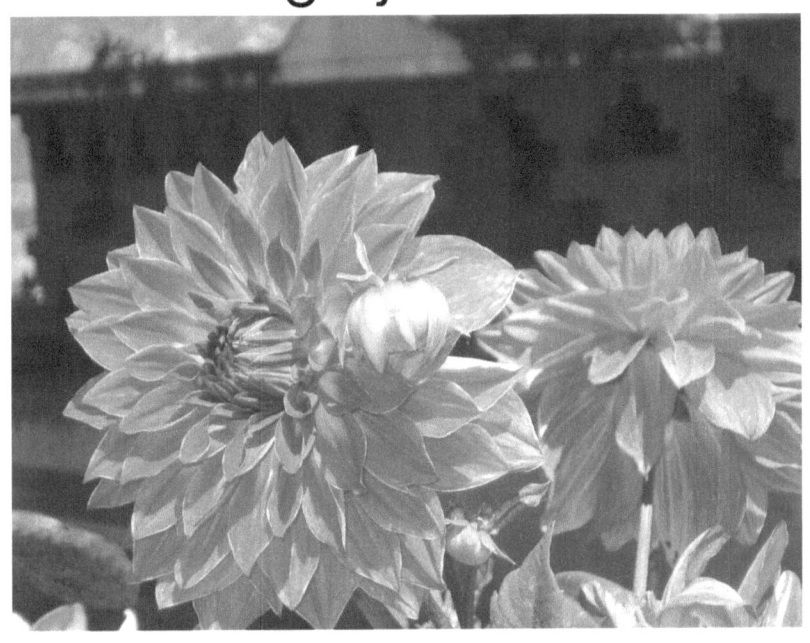

Dahlias from Kopan Monastery, Nepal

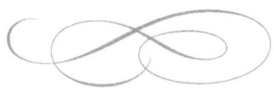

It appears that yoga is the cure-all for everything. What's up with that? It's the combination of the mind, body, and spirit working together. Western medicine does not address all three parts of our being, it only addresses the Body. Many of us in the west have been trained to think of alleviating a symptom, and not the problem. Yesterday I told my husband I had a headache, his quick reply was *"Get rid of it, take and Advil"*. My response was, *"I want to know what is causing the headache and get rid of <u>that</u> instead"*. I pulled out my yoga mat and got into Ado Mukha Svanasana (Down Dog). The tightness in my lower back was relieved, my calves got a great stretch, I let my head wobble around releasing tension around my neck, and three minutes later my headache was gone. Yes, yoga is the cure-all.

There's a book with research funded by the National Institute of Health which details a program for reversing heart disease. The program has 13 years of research behind it, and I quote a summary statement from the author, Dr. Dean Ornish[18], *"All techniques derive from*

---

18 http://www.ornishspectrum.com - Dr. Dean Ornish Preventive Medicine Research Institute

yoga". Dean Michael Ornish is a the president and founder of the Preventive Medicine Research Institute in Sausalito, California. He is also a Clinical Professor of Medicine at the University of California, San Francisco. Ornish highlights yoga's techniques in breathing, stretching, and mindfulness to reduce stress and heal the whole person versus just the illness. Other examples include Dr. Carl and Stephanie Simonton who offer programs for cancer patients worldwide[19]. Dr. Carl who passed away in 2009 was know as the father of mind-body medicine for cancer patients. The center still offers services from the West Coast to South Africa! The focus for patients is training in relaxation and mental imagery for general health. The Simonton method includes the whole person, not just getting rid of symptoms—how beliefs, attitudes, lifestyle choices, spiritual and psychological perspectives can affect our health and even the course of our disease. Lastly, the Lamaze Method of breathing for childbirth is not used as much as in the past decades. Guess what today's doctors and the Mayo Clinic often suggest? Prenatal Yoga and Yoga for Childbirth classes.

So we've covered childbirth, cancer, and heart disease. Let me touch on other benefits of yoga. Our equilibrium can become a little 'off' due to muscles being overworked over a period of time contributing to loss of balance. Yoga is about posture and many poses strengthen the ankles as well as balance the muscles that have been strained causing our imbalanced posture. Yoga improves the

[19] http://www.simontoncenter.com - The Simonton Center for Cancer Patients

quality of our sleep, it helps us find the *'off switch'* for our minds leading to a deeper rest. Yoga postures, particularly twists, aid the natural flow of our digestive system relieving constipation and other intestinal issues. Yoga helps the endocrine, vascular, musculature and nervous systems which supports steady metabolism, mental clarity, emotional calmness and relief of typical aches and pains. The breathing in Yoga (Pranayama), increases O2 in the bloodstream which stimulates the heart while reducing tension and stress. Do teachers still tell kids to take three deep breaths before explaining that horrible thing that happened on the playground? They should!

Age is not a barrier for Yoga. The low impact style of practice is safe for older students, and the mindfulness of the practice is great for children. The fact that the only equipment needed is a Yoga Mat makes it accessible to nearly everyone. And even ten minutes a day of yoga will prove a benefit to your health and overall wellbeing. I ran programs for children over two years at the Boys & Girls Clubs in San Francisco. During that time, many children in the program who were labeled ADD (Attention Deficit Disorder) were noted to have better grades and a calmer home life. Most of the little darlings who practiced with me could not wait for the weekly class, as if their mind, body, and spirit were crying out for the yoga experience. My private clients are mostly between the ages of 50 and 75, many who suffer from some type of illness or degradation of health. And I am honored to serve them all. One student cried at the end of the first class, as she realized she was sitting cross legged after coming out of savasana. She suffers chronic arthritis in both knees and had not been able to bend them in this way in years.

As a Bhakti Yogi, I've worked with double hip replacements, scoliosis, hypertension, heart disease, plantar fasciitis, cancer rehab & healing, epilepsy, stroke rehab, fused bones, polio therapy, war veterans, AIDS survivors, and those with mystery illnesses. Somehow, those in need find me. Perhaps their spirits intuit my deep compassion. And though it seems as if I heal them, the unconditional love and gentle guidance I give leads them to heal themselves.

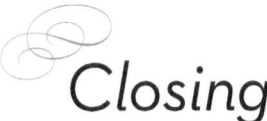

Closing

In closing, I sincerely hope I have fed you well with information on Bhakti. As a Messenger from God, I pray that my words have reached your heart with the purity of spirit from the Divine.

Living a Bhakti Life is not for everyone, we are all different. It is a choice that is born in the heart and developed through your life journey. Take from this book what fills your soul and leave behind what is not needed. Meditate on the things that need clarity, or contact me through letters or the website. We can all live the Bhakti Life, even if only a little bit at a time if we just surrender to what is.

You are welcome to study more with me on retreats, as I offer them each year. I am also available to bring retreat trainings directly to you as a private group.

Nature is a part of Bhakti and many of my retreats require you to leave the comforts of home to help you grow spiritually. Combined with my teachings, my retreats will help you reach the next level of understanding, compassion, and unconditional love.

Join me.

www.yogaofdevotion.org

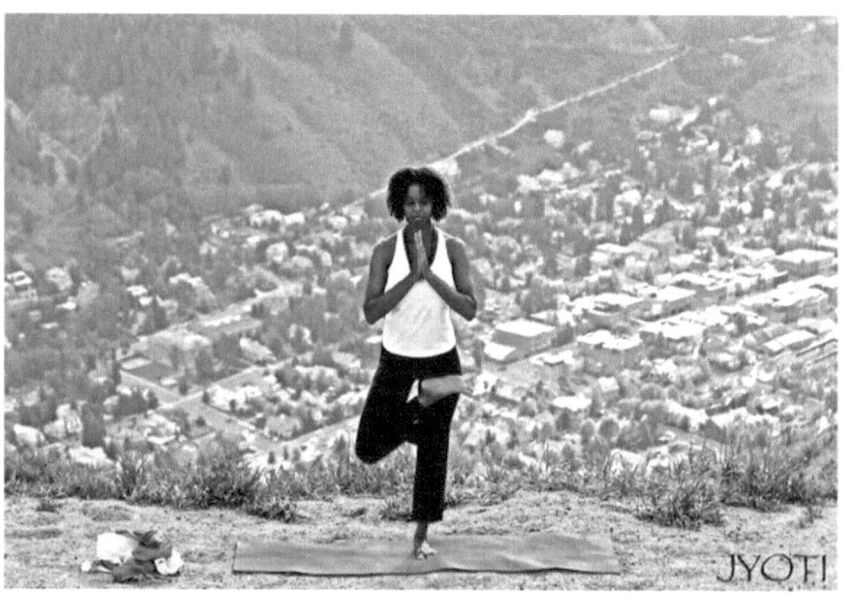

Appendix:
List of Bhakti Asana Postures

Some photos not available

1. Chakravakasana (Cat-Cow)
    I will watch the flexibility of my ego today, aware that
    it causes bends & turns in my journey

2. Matsyndrasana (Seated Twist)
    Twisting left, I look back at where I've come from,
    accepting and releasing all. Twisting right, I look at
    where I'm going, visualizing my future

3. Utpluti (Lotus off the ground)
    Even with the entanglements of life, I will rise above.

4.   Tadasana (Mountain Pose)
     I stand tall in the majesty of the Divine, presenting
     myself as an expression of life

5.   Surya Namaskara (Sun Salutation)
     I take in all the experiences of my life -good and bad,
     and gracefully swan dive into this day

6.   Uttanasana (Forward Bend)
     I will be flexible with others today

7.   Uttanasana on Toes
     I will raise my consciousness today, functioning on a
     higher level of flexibility

8.   Plank
     I will hold myself up in the face of adversity

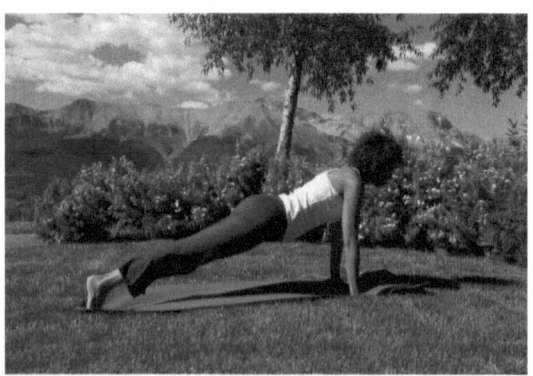

9. Chaturanga Dandasana

    I will Lower my expectations of others

10. Urdva Mukha Svanasana

    I push through it all and look up to the Divine for my power and strength

11. Adho Mukha Svanasana

    I can find my balance; half weight on my hands and half in my legs = rest, and I can find the balance in my life

12. Virabhadrasana I

    I am the warrior of my life, I co-create each day holding my intentions up to the Divine

13. Virabhadrasana II

    I am the warrior of my life, the past behind me and pointing towards my future. Although I know my direction, I am open (chest and back) to others suggestions

14. Virabhadrasana III

    I take all my gifts into my heart, and move forward to share them with the world

15. <u>Trikonasana</u>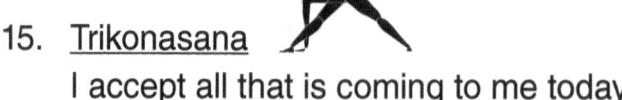
    I accept all that is coming to me today

16. <u>Parivritti Trikonasana</u>
    I accept all that occurred yesterday

17. <u>Uttita Parsvakonasana</u>
    I will reach for new ways of thinking & being

18. <u>Ardha Chandrasana</u> (Half Moon)
    I can soar through this life with grace and ease. One
    day my Spirit will fly away with the Divine

19. <u>Garudhasana</u> (Eagle)
    Though life may twist me up, I drop all my burdens
    at the feet of the Divine, and rise up untangled and
    Free as a Bird.

20. <u>Vasisthasana</u> (Side Plank)
    I give myself freely to the Divine, my strengths and
    vulnerabilities

21. <u>Parivritti Vasisthasana</u> (Wild Thang)
    I completely Surrender my heart to the Divine

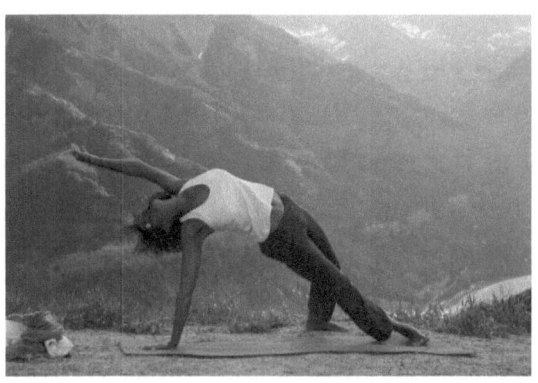

22. <u>Vrksasana</u> (Tree Pose)
    May I be grounded today in who I really am, May I find
    creativity & sexuality in my experiences today, May
    I watch my ego today – that it not get out of control,
    May I swing up to my heart – allowing it to guide my
    actions today, May I guard my words today – that they
    may be sweet or non existent, May I trust my Intuition
    today – my direct communication with my true self,
    May the Divine fill my crown with Love and Light –
    that I may operate on a higher level of consciousness
    today, and May I always express my gratitude to the
    one source that gives me life.

23. <u>Navasana</u> (Boat Pose)
    I can hold it up for the Divine, who has held me up so
    many times in my life

24. <u>Purvatanasna</u> (Up plank)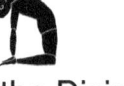
Every Valley Shall be Exhalted!

25. <u>Eka Pada Raja Kapotasana</u>
I release all that I have done to hurt others, and all the hurts done unto me. I scoop up the forgiveness that is before me, raising it over my head and bathing myself in that forgiveness.

26. <u>Virasana</u> (Hero)
The Hero is within you. Find it, and begin to co-create your life.

27. <u>Ustrasana</u> (Camel)
I open my heart, that the Divine may fill me with light for the day

28. <u>Urdhva Dhanurasana</u> (Wheel)
I exhault my mind, body, spirit, and whole constitution to the Divine, opening my heart to lift up others to the Divine Light

29. <u>Halasana</u> (Plow)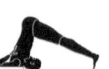
I will bend over backwards for someone else today

30. Nirlamba Sarvangasana
    (Unsupported Shoulderstand)
    No path is ever completely straight, there's always an
    angle of support. The Divine is that support.

31. Salamba Sarvangasana
    (Supported Shoulderstand)
    No path is ever completely straight, the angle of
    support is with you, as close to me as my hands.

32. Urdhva Padmasana (Shoulderstand in Lotus)
    I can flow with life's twists, lifting them up to the Divine
    for guidance

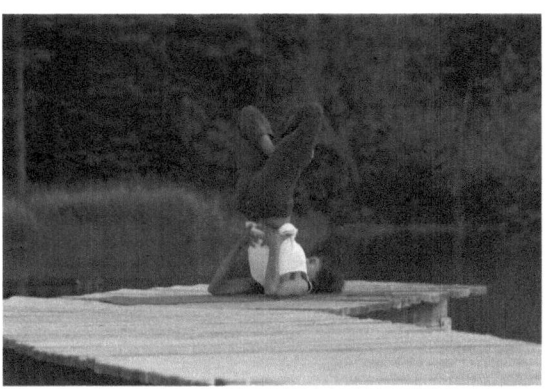

33. <u>Parsva Padmasana in Sarvangasana</u> (Twisted Lotus in Shoulderstand)
I offer my ego, which causes these twists, to the Divine for purification

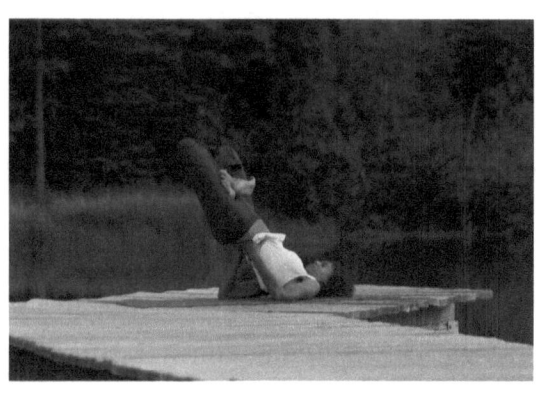

34. <u>Sirsasana (Headstand)</u>
I can view things from someone else's perspective, completely unlike mine.

35. <u>Adho Mukha Vriksasana</u> (Handstand)
I exhalt myself to the Divine, in complete trust that you are with me.

36. <u>Balasana</u> (Child's Pose)
I am but a child, still learning to play nicely in this universe. Please guide me.

37. <u>Jathara Parivritti</u>

I lay often in a paradox, twisting towards one path while my higher self yearns for the opposite path. I relax now and let it all go.

38. <u>Savasana</u>

I will Work & Rest with equal intensity. I will surrender it all now - This is my gift to myself.

39. <u>Bhaktasana</u>

I surrender everything unto the Divine and do all in your name.

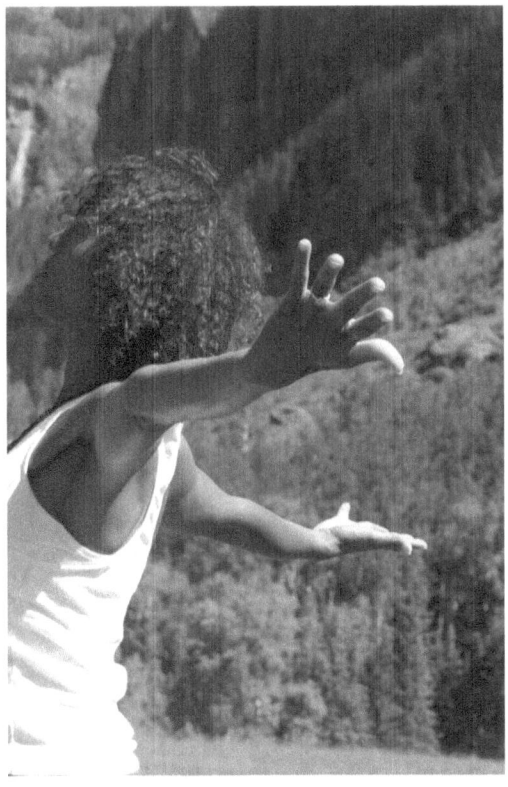

Notes

Yoga of Devotion is a non-profit 501(c)(3) registered under Telluride Flights Worldwide Children's Relief Fund since 2007. Since The Bhakti Asana practice was a gift from above, Angela decided at the inception of her business to continue sharing the gift through Retreats, Humanitarian Work, and proceeds.

The purchase of this book or any products from Yoga of Devotion help children in need around the world, and are tax deductible for you. Materials available on the website include DVD's on Bhakti Yoga instruction. CD's are available on Meditation, Ayurveda & Yoga, Chanting, and Meditations for Chemotherapy. Visit the website to purchase or contact the office at the address below.

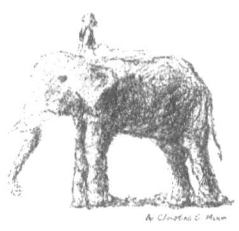

Bhakti Asana - Yoga of Devotion

Retreats are offered two-four times a year and are also tax deducible. Seva is a part of every retreat. Visit the website for upcoming trips. Angela is also available for custom retreats created just for your group!

Yoga of Devotion also offers a Stress Relief App: 'Stress Relief with Yoga of Devotion' available for download at the Apple iTunes store for iPhone, iPad and iPod. Also available for Droid phones in the Google for Droid App Store.

<u>If you would like to make a donation, visit the website or mail to</u>:

Yoga of Devotion
One Embarcadero Center, Suite #500
San Francisco, CA 94111
www.yogaofdevotion.org
415.623.2088

Thank you!

Yoga of Devotion has supported and/or personally served:

- IDEP Foundation for Children & Families - Bali, Indonesia During Jakarta Quake and Volcano

- Casa de Milagros Orphanage - Sacred Valley, Peru Mother's Day Visit

- Hamilton Shelter - San Francisco, California Children's Empowerment Program

- Maasai Joy School - Arusha, Tanzania Organic Garden, Affirmation Wall of Hope & Thanksgiving Feast

- Sydney Children's Hospital - Sydney, Australia Children's Play Program + Children's book for Wellness

- Dubai Cares - Dubai, UAE Global Citizen Program for Children & Teens

- Work to Ride - Philadelphia, Pennsylvania Equestrian/Polo program for Teens at risk

- dZi Foundation - Kathmandu, Nepal Humanitarian projects for Rural Villages

- Glide Foundation - San Francisco, California Spiritual Yoga for the Glide Community & Homeless Bagging for 700 lunch program for the Homeless

- Invisible Children - Uganda, Africa Empowerment & Freedom of Child Soldiers

- Left to Tell Orphanage - Rwanda, Africa Safety and Shelter for Orphans left from Genocide

- Yoga for Hope - San Francisco, California Fundraiser for Cancer Patients

- UCSF Hellen Diller Cancer Center - San Francisco, California Lecture Presentation: Spring Wellness Day

- San Francisco City Departments - San Francisco, California Contracted to provide Stress Relief for Employees Ambassador Program

- San Francisco Foster Care Wellness - San Francisco, California Presentation for parents and children in Foster Care

- The Boys & Girls Club - San Francisco, California Kids Crossing Cultures Program (Nepal, India, Peru)

- Willowcreek Academy - Sausalito, California Kids Crossing Cultures Program (Nepal)

- Grattan Elementary - San Francisco, California Kids Crossing Cultures Program (India)

- Mercy & Grace Orphanage - Andhra Pradesh, India Dream Big Pillow Program, and Child Empowerment Untouchables Sewing Program - Vijayawada, India

- Dubai Yoga & Music Fest for International Peace Gathering in the safest region of the Mid East Promoting Peace

- Evolve Yoga Festival - Sydney & Melbourne, Australia Adult Empowerment & Bhakti

- Telluride Yoga Festival - Telluride, Colorado Community / Intentional Visioning & Empowerment

- Itahari Villge Hospital - Itahari, Nepal Kids Crossing Cultures Program

- YogaFest - Brisbane, Australia Community Bhakti & Surrender

- From Hand to Hand - Kenya, Africa Organic farming, training for sustainability in Africa Empowerment for Women & Children Co-venture with Swami Padmapadananda, of Sivananda

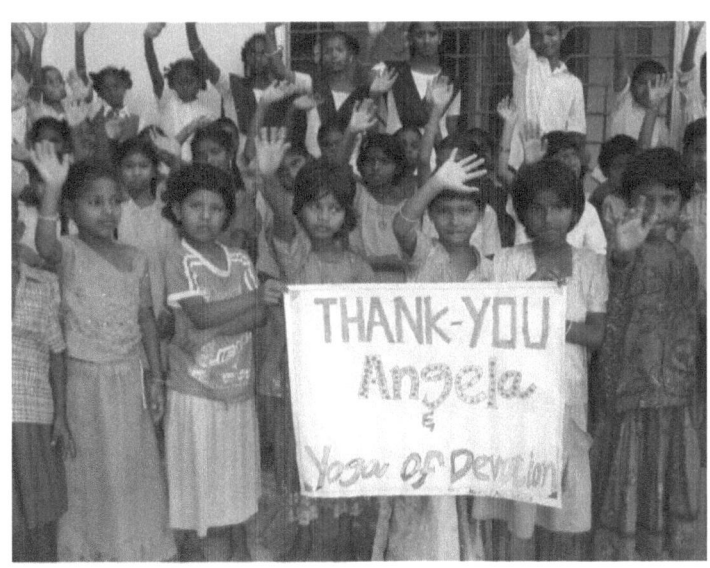

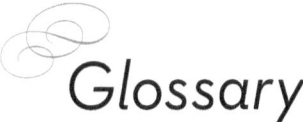

Glossary

A

Ahimsa: A term meaning to do no harm (literally: the avoidance of violence – himsa).

Affirmation: 1. The act of affirming or the state of being affirmed; assertion. 2. Something declared to be true; a positive statement or judgment.

Anjali Mudra: Añjali Mudrā or Pranamasana is a hand gesture which is practiced throughout Asia. It is used as a sign of respect and a greeting in India and amongst yoga practitioners and adherents of similar traditions. The gesture is incorporated into many yoga asanas. Hands are held together at the heart as in prayer.

Anterior Fontanelle: A diamond-shaped unossified area between the frontal and two parietal bones just above an infant's forehead at the junction of the coronal and sagittal sutures, also called the soft spot.

Asana:is a body position, typically associated with the practice of Yoga

Atman: The individual soul or essence or the essence that is eternal, unchanging, and indistinguishable from the essence of the universe.

$\mathcal{B}$

Bhakti: In Hinduism and Buddhism it is religious devotion in the form of active involvement of a devotee in worship of the divine. Within monotheistic Hinduism, it is the love felt by the worshipper towards the personal God

Brahman: a Hindu of the highest caste traditionally assigned to the priesthood

C

Chakra: The concept of chakra features in tantric and yogic traditions of Hinduism and Buddhism. Chakra are believed to be centers of the body from which a person can collect energy. They are connected to major organs or glands that govern other body parts.

Coronal Suture: The line of junction of the frontal bone with the two parietal bones.

D

Dhyana: meditation, one of the eight limbs or paths of Patanjalis yoga, aimed at self-realization and self-knowledge. When the mind is no longer distracted from the object of concentration, then dhyana is realized

Divine: of, relating to, or proceeding directly from God or a God

E

Eight Limbs of Ashtanga: Ashtanga yoga literally means "8 limbs yoga. " These limbs are defined in the the second chapter of the Yoga Sutras of Patanjali.

The following are the 8 practices or limbs:

1. yama (moral restraints) – how we relate to others

2. niyama (observances) – how we relate to ourselves

3. āsana (posture) – how we relate to our body

4. prānāyāma (breath extension) – how we relate to our breath or spirit

5. pratyāhāra (sensory withdrawal) – how we relate to our sense organs

6. dhāranā (concentration) – how we relate to our mind

7. dhyāna (meditation) – moving beyond the mind

8. samādhi (meditative absorption) – deep realization and inner union

F

Frontal Lobe: One of the main structural divisions of the brain, which is located, as it is implied by its name, in the front part of the brain. The frontal lobe performs several important brain functions including planning and carrying out movements, judgment, insight, language, personality, and emotional control, among others.

G

Gayatri Mantra:The word mantra is Sanskrit and it means: syllable(s) or sacred word(s). Mantras are vibrational formulas that are recited silently within, or spoken, or sung outwardly. There are mantras in Sanskrit as well as Japanese, Chinese and Tibetan languages. Gayatri Mantra is one in particular.

Guru: a Sanskrit term for "teacher" or "master", especially in Indian religions

H

Higher Purpose: The way that the 'higher purpose' is typically used is to find something that the person will accept as being of greater importance than themselves. This then may be used as a lever, framing decisions that the person has to make in terms of a choice between the higher purpose and themselves.

I

Interfaith: Of, relating to, or involving persons of different religious faiths

Ishvara: A philosophical concept in Hinduism, meaning controller or God

Ishvarapranidhana: Ishvarapranidhana represents surrender to, and love for, the divinity within the individual in Hinduism and Yoga

J

Jivamukti: An enlightened being of the highest order. Liberated from stress and worry.

K

Karma Cycle: The concept of "action" or "deed", understood as that which causes the entire cycle of cause and effect. In other words, you get what you put into life and vice versa.

Kundalini: literally means coiled. In yoga, a "corporeal energy"[1] - an unconscious, instinctive or libidinal force or Shakti, lies coiled at the base of the spine. kundalini awakening results in deep meditation, enlightenment and bliss

M

Meditation: Private religious devotion or mental exercise, in which techniques of concentration and contemplation are used to reach a heightened level of spiritual awareness.

Walking Meditation: Same as above walking at a slow mindful pace.

O

Occipital Lobe: The visual processing center of the mammalian brain located on the medial side of the occipital lobe

Olfactory Center: The part of the brain responsible for the subjective appreciation of odors, a complex group of neurons located near the junction of the temporal and parietal lobes.

Oxytocin: A hormone made in the brain that plays a role in childbirth and lactation by causing muscles to contract in the uterus (womb) and the mammary glands in the breast. Animal studies have shown that oxytocin also has a role in pair bonding, mate-guarding, and social memory

$\mathcal{P}$

Patanjali: Flourished late 2nd century b.c., Indian scholar and philosopher: sometimes regarded as the founder of yoga.

Perusha: Male en-ergy, one of the two manifestations of cosmic consciousness; an energy that has passive awareness but is without form or attribute

Prakriti:Prakriti is material nature in its germinal state, eternal and beyond perception. When it comes into contact with the soul or self (purusha), it starts a process of evolution that leads through several stages to the creation of the existing material world

Prana: The life force or vital energy, which permeates the body

Pranayama: A Sanskrit word meaning "extension of the prā□a or breath" or more accurately, "extension of the life force"

Puja: In Hinduism, the term puja refers to the worship of deities. Such worship can take one of three forms in Hinduism: temple worship, domestic worship and communal worship.

S

Saggital Suture: the serrated connection between the two parietal bones of the skull, coursing down the midline from the coronal suture to the upper part of the lambdoidal suture.

Samadhi: The highest stage in meditation, in which a person experiences oneness with the universe.

Samsara: The Sanskrit word samsara means "journeying." In Buddhism, as well as in Hinduism and Jainism, samsara is defined as a cycle of birth, death, and rebirth.

Sanskrit: (Linguistics / Languages) an ancient language of India, the language of the Vedas, of Hinduism, and of an extensive philosophical and scientific literature dating from the beginning of the first millennium bc It is the oldest recorded member of the Indic branch of the Indo-European family of languages

Santosha: When we can be satisfied with our circumstances and with what we have and are, we experience contentment and Santosha.

Self Realization: Self-realization is an expression used in psychology, spirituality and Eastern religions. The basic premise of self-realization is that there exists an authentic self which has to be discovered by psychological or spiritual self-striving. Self-realization can be a gradual or instantaneous phenomena depending on the school of thought but in all cases it involves extensive preparation of mind and emotions to recognize self-realization when it occurs.

Seva: Seva means service. In Sikhism, seva refers to selfless service for altruistic purposes on behalf of, and for the betterment of a Community.

Surya Namaskar: ancient Indian yogic exercise, ("salutation to the Sun"), which is a combination of 12 positions performed sequentially

Sutra: In Hinduism, a brief aphoristic composition; in Buddhism, a more extended exposition of a subject and the basic form of the scripture

Transcellular fluids: A body fluid that is not inside cells but is separated from plasma and interstitial fluid by cellular barriers.

U

Upanishads: a collection of philosophical texts which form the theoretical basis for the Hindu religion.

V

Vedic Texts: the most ancient memorials of Indian literature, created in the period from the end of the second millennium to the first half of the first millennium B.C. in the ancient Indian language of Vedic.

Y

Yoga: commonly known generic term for physical, mental, and spiritual disciplines which originated in ancient India

Yogini: The feminine form of yogi

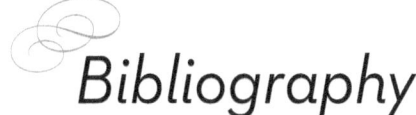

Bibliography

[1] Medicine Plus www.nlm.nih.gov

[2] Adam Medical Images www.adameducation.com

[3] www.answers.com/topic/suture

[4] Sūtra (Sanskrit: सूत्र sūtra, Devanagari: , Pāli: sutta), literally means a thread or line that holds things together, and more metaphorically refers to an aphorism (or line, rule, formula),

[5] The Yoga Sutras of Patanjali, Translation by Sri Swami Satchidananada 1978

[6] The Yoga Sutras of Patanjali, Pg.150 lower 4th paragraph

[7] Bhagavad Gita Chapter 18 By this same love and worship doth he know Me as I am, how high and wonderful, And knowing, straightway enters into Me. And whatsoever deeds he doeth-fixed In Me, as in his refuge - he hath won For ever and for ever by My grace Th' Eternal Rest! So win thou! In thy thoughts Do all thou dost for Me! Renounce for Me! Sacrifice heart and mind and will to Me!

[8] Bhagavad Gita Chapter 11, Shloks (verses) 53-55 after exhibiting His cosmic form, "It is not possible to see me as you have done through the study of the Vedas or by austerities or gifts or by sacrifice; it is only by one-pointed devotion (Bhakti) to me and me alone that you thus see and know

me as I am in reality and ultimately reach me. It is he alone who dedicates all his notions and actions to me with a knowledge of my superiority, my devotee with no attachment and who has no enmity to any living being that can reach me". Bhakti therefore, is the only way to the true knowledge of God and the surest way to reach Him. **Bhakti: Unwavering Devotion & Love for God**

[9] http://www.swamisatchidananda.org/docs2/home.htm

[10] International Sai Organization www.sathyasai.org

[11] Faith Rivera – "Child of this Universe" Lil' Girl Productions / Spiritual Songstress & Writer

[12] Richard Hooper, 2007 – The Teachings of Four Mystical Traditions; Jesus, Buddha, Krishna, & Lao Tzu / Sanctuary Publications

[13] Pg. 22, Armageddon in Retrospect, Kurt Vonnegut 2008

[14] http://online.sfsu.edu/~rone/Buddhism/footsteps.htm

[15] The Mind of Jesus, pg.7, William Barclay, Harper & Row Publishers, New York 1961

[16] The Bhagavad Gita, Translated by Sir Edwin Arnold, Ch.13 pg.139, Watkins Publishing, London 2006

[17] http://www.pbs.org/wnet/religionandethics/episodes/july-17-2009/faith-and-the-brain/3597/ - Dr. Andrew Newberg - University of Pennsylvania Brain Study

[18] http://www.ornishspectrum.com - Dr. Dean Ornish Preventive Medicine Research Institute

[19] http://www.simontoncenter.com - The Simonton Center for Cancer Patients

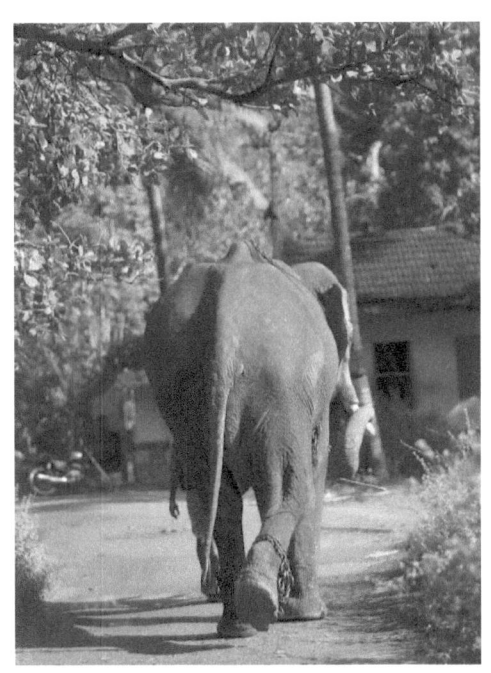

The End

www.ingramcontent.com/pod-product-compliance
Lightning Source LLC
Chambersburg PA
CBHW051422280526
45785CB00003B/1118